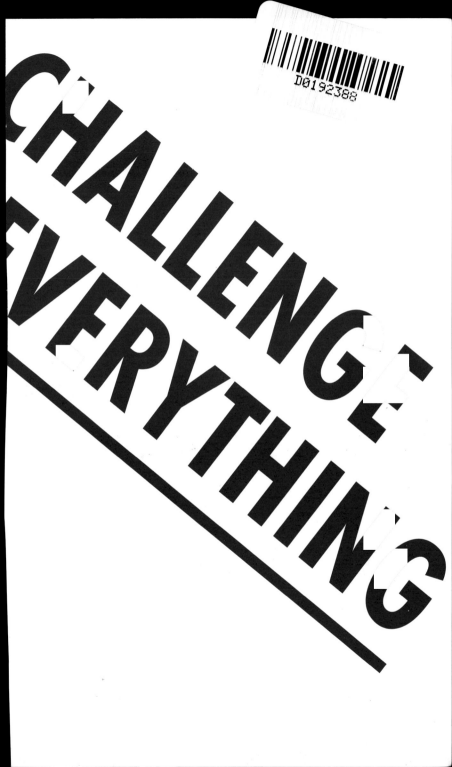

First published in the UK in 2020 by
Pavilion Books Company Limited
43 Great Ormond Street
London, WC1N 3HZ

Design: Ben Peppiatt pages 94, 98;
Arthur Stovell pages 31, 88, 94;
Jo Wheeler page 94; Ollie Whittall page 94.

Graphics: Clive Russell front cover, back cover, pages 07, 49, 88, 144.

Wood-cuts: Miles Glyn cover spine, pages 04, 05, 08, 15, 17, 44,
45, 62, 63, 68, 76, 104, 115, 118, 128, 133.

Publisher: Neil Dunnicliffe

Editorial Advisor: Stella Gurney

Editorial Reviewer: Alice Corrie

Editor: Hattie Grylls

Designer: Sarah Crookes

ISBN: 9781843654643

A CIP catalogue record for this book is available from the British Library.

10 9 8 7 6 5 4 3 2 1

Printed by CPI Group (UK) Ltd.

This book can be ordered at www.pavilionbooks.com, or try your local bookshop.

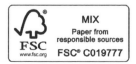

MIX
Paper from
responsible sources
FSC® C019777

BLUE SANDFORD

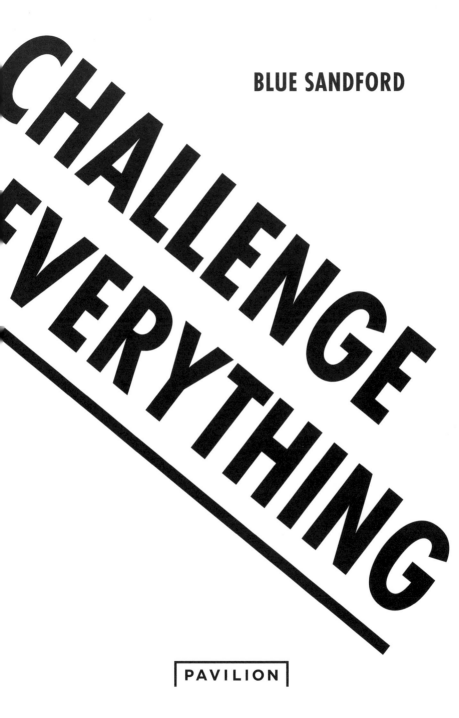

CHALLENGE EVERYTHING

PAVILION

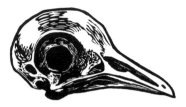

CONTENTS

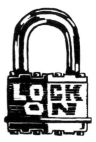

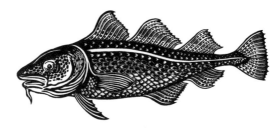

INTRO

When my publishers first approached me about writing this book, I had to think carefully. I'm one of the coordinators for Extinction Rebellion Youth London and my primary aim in life is to draw attention to climate change and make the planet cleaner and greener. But the world does not need yet another case of 'greenwashing' or 'virtue signalling': phrases that mean appearing to make efforts to cut your carbon footprint without actually achieving anything of substance.

In my research I came across so many awful examples of this. One of the most ridiculous was a blog that recommended the use of e-tickets for aeroplane flights to avoid wasting paper – as if this could somehow balance out the pollution of the flight itself! It made me laugh and then want to cry... I was worried that this book might go the same way: that readers would feel they'd 'done their bit' just by buying or reading it, without anyone having really changed their behaviour. In this way, I felt that maybe it could even do more harm than good.

Often, greenwashing is unintentional. People put all their efforts into small well-known things like recycling, while overlooking different changes that wouldn't take a lot more effort but would have a much bigger impact. Of course, every little helps and I don't want to be dismissive about anything that's a step in the right direction.

Recycle, compost, bring your own bag, cycle, walk, don't take cabs, make eco bricks (if you don't know about these, look them up!), turn down the heating and air conditioning, turn off the lights, turn off the tap, use a refillable water bottle, use a menstrual cup, don't fill up the kettle, use ecosia as your search engine, buy local, etc, etc.

These things are important, especially if we all do them, but they can sometimes just absolve guilt and give people a justification to carry on living carbon-intensive lives without really challenging themselves.

After a lot of thought, I decided that I can't take responsibility for whether people read this book and then do nothing. That responsibility lies with YOU. Every small choice we make as individuals can add up when an army of people make the same decisions. But also think about the actions that will get the biggest and best results.

And don't take things for granted – CHALLENGE EVERYTHING. That means challenging big business and your government and, most of all, challenging yourself to act now and save the planet.

I hope you enjoy this book. I hope it makes you think, and I hope it makes you want to challenge the status quo, change the world and save all our lives.

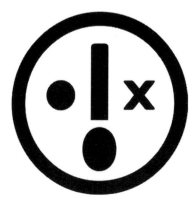

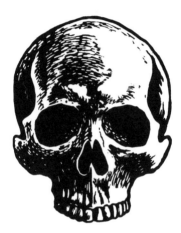

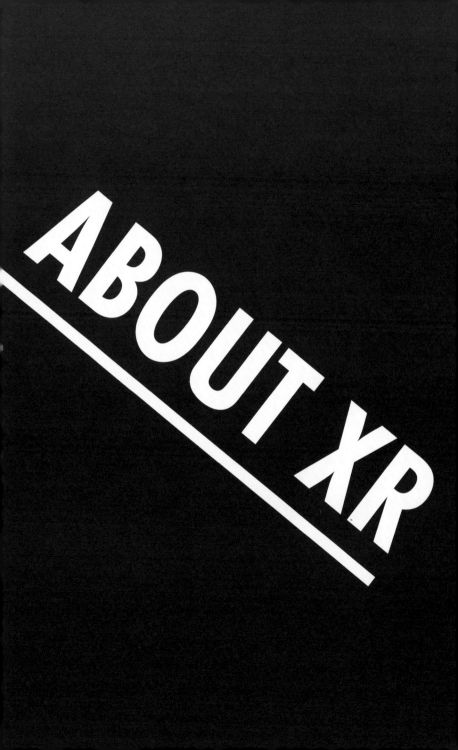

ABOUT XR

WE ARE A GENERATION
THAT HAS NEVER KNOWN
A STABLE CLIMATE AND
THAT WILL BE DEFINED
BY HOW THE WORLD
RESPONDS TO THE CLIMATE
AND ECOLOGICAL CRISIS.

XR YOUTH

Extinction Rebellion (XR) is an international apolitical movement that uses non-violent direct action and civil disobedience in an attempt to persuade governments to act on the Climate and Ecological Emergency, halt mass extinction and minimise the risk of social collapse.

XR was launched in the UK in October 2018 by Roger Hallam and Gail Bradbrook, along with other activists. In November 2018, five bridges across the River Thames in London were blocked in the first large-scale action. In April 2019 the group held its first large demonstration in London. Over 11 days, many of the city's busiest areas were brought to a standstill. Over a thousand non-violent protesters were arrested for disruption.

Since this first major action, the movement has grown very quickly. There are now about 130 Extinction Rebellion groups across the UK and more all around the world. In October 2019 XR held the International Rebellion, with disruption occurring in the UK, the US, Germany, Australia, Belgium, Spain, New Zealand, Holland, France, Austria and elsewhere.

XR AIMS & PRINCIPLES

XR is by its nature decentralised. Anybody who believes in the three core aims, and follows the ten principles, can act in the name of XR:

AIMS

TELL THE TRUTH
Government must tell the truth by declaring a climate and ecological emergency, working with other institutions to communicate the urgency for change.

ACT NOW
Government must act now to halt biodiversity loss and reduce greenhouse gas emissions to net zero by 2025.

BEYOND POLITICS
Government must create, and be led by the decisions of, a citizens' assembly on climate and ecological justice.

PRINCIPLES

1

We have a shared vision of change – creating a world that is fit for generations to come.

2

We set our mission on what is necessary – mobilising 3.5% of the population to achieve system change by using ideas such as 'momentum-driven organising' to achieve this.

3

We need a regenerative culture – creating a culture that is healthy, resilient, and adaptable.

4

We openly challenge ourselves and this toxic system, leaving our comfort zones to take action for change.

5

We value reflecting and learning, following a cycle of action, reflection, learning, and planning for more action (learning from other movements and contexts as well as our own experiences).

6

We welcome everyone and every part of everyone – working actively to create safer and more accessible spaces.

7

We actively mitigate for power – breaking down hierarchies of power for more equitable participation.

8

We avoid blaming and shaming – we live in a toxic system, but no one individual is to blame.

9

We are a non-violent network using non-violent strategy and tactics as the most effective way to bring about change.

10

We are based on autonomy and decentralisation – we collectively create the structures we need to challenge power.

ROLES WITHIN XR

Much of XR's media coverage is focused on mass arrest. Many XR members accept the possibility of arrest and imprisonment at an action, but this is not a necessity to join the movement.

Those that do allow themselves to be arrested or imprisoned do it to highlight the inadequacy of a system that incriminates those fighting against loss of biodiversity and human suffering.

It also follows in the tradition of many grassroots campaigns such as the Suffragettes and the civil rights movements. Arrestees are supported by an Arrest Welfare Team and a Legal Team.

There are many ways to help out the cause that do not involve being arrested. Local XR groups are committed to finding a role for every keen supporter, through an Affinity Group. Every skill is welcomed – writers, lawyers, designers, artists, musicians, builders, cooks, cleaners, counsellors and more.

You can also support those in the middle of an Action by bringing them food, opening your homes to people who are not local, or making phone calls to the community through the group Rebel Ringers.

XR YOUTH

There are many community groups within XR that are related to a shared self-identity, for example, faith, profession, ethnicity, age or sexual identity.

XR Youth is the young voice of the rebellion, a network for everyone born after 1990. It is also one of the biggest groups, with at least 80 XR Youth sub-groups throughout the world.

XR Youth recognises that the broader movement isn't perfect and that some of their priorities are different. This is because we are fighting for our own future, as well as the future of our children. We are the generation that has never known a stable climate.

We emphasise climate justice for indigenous groups and those in the global south who are on the frontline of the climate crisis. You can read this in our Truths.

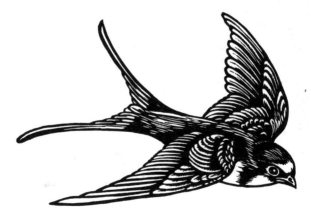

THE XR YOUTH TRUTHS

THE TRUTH IS our demands are not enough.

The urgency of the climate crisis requires a just response centred on human rights, equity and justice.

The way our world currently looks is built on exploitation.

We need to transform the world in order to prevent further climate catastrophe.

We need to transform the way we live in order for us to survive.

A just transition recognises that the way we transform must include changes that restore the balance of power and give power and resources back to those people who have had them taken away.

THE TRUTH IS the only solution to the climate crisis is to restore and repair land, re-unite people with their homelands and work to transform our relationship with each other and our planet.

THE TRUTH IS communities of colour, migrant communities and working-class communities bear the brunt of the climate crisis. These communities, even in wealthy countries, lack the resources due to an ingrained system of classism and racism.

THE TRUTH IS the ideology that has created the hostile environment for migrants is the same ideology that has created a hostile climate worldwide.

THE TRUTH IS that we have exploited world resources and caused climate chaos.

Many people are migrating to find the safety that has been taken away from them, many have been settled for decades building the relative safety we enjoy now.

THE TRUTH IS competing for resources is not the answer, either inside or beyond our borders. We need to work to repair the damage to people and planet and manage resources collectively for all.

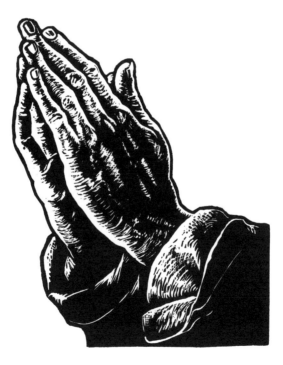

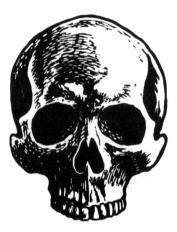

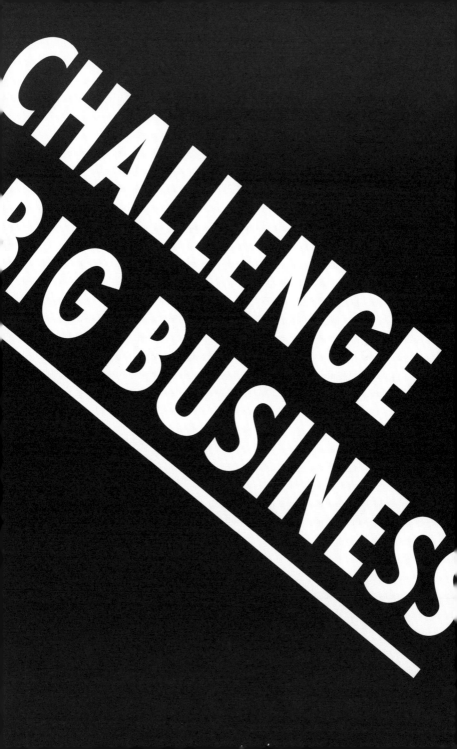

A lot of environmental devastation can be traced back to many corporations not caring about sustainability or the pollution from factories and power stations. These businesses aren't being held accountable for the damage they're doing to our planet.

Big businesses have a lot of power, because much of our world runs according to whoever has the most money – and they have a lot. This power could be used to change things for the better, both from the inside – becoming more ethical and eco-friendly in their production processes and practices – and also in the influence they have with politicians, the media and other big companies.

So how can you make big businesses want to wield their power in the right direction? You could begin by writing to the owner or main decision-maker, the Chief Executive Officer (CEO – you can find out who they are and their contact details online), explaining the dangers of the climate crisis and the role their business has in it. You could ask whether they are parents and highlight how their children will suffer just as much as the rest of our generation. You could communicate with the workers about the dangers of the climate crisis and ask them to put pressure on the company from the inside.

It's possible that when they understand that their customers care about the climate crisis, businesses will want to do something about it, even if only to make sure that people will like their image and carry on buying things from them. But while these things would be great, they're hard to achieve by subtle persuasion. The simplest way to get businesses to change their behaviour is to disrupt their sales – and therefore their profits – and the easiest (and most legal) way to do this is by boycotting them. Single out a brand or a specific product and refuse to buy it.

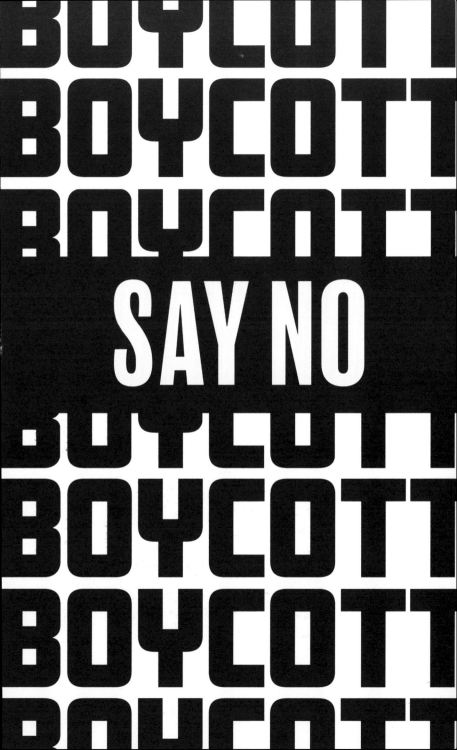

Boycotting has a long and successful history in social movements, most famously in the civil rights movements of the USA. In the Montgomery bus boycott of 1955 and '56, African American people (including Rosa Parks) refused to use the city's buses because of their segregated seating. The boycott lasted for 381 days and attracted so much interest all over the country that eventually the case was taken to court and the civil rights movement won.

Boycotting is effective, and it's also something easy that you can persuade others to do: your friends, your class, even the school. What's more, it's a media-friendly story that'll show you in a good light. You're the good guy, taking a stand, and you're not disrupting or inconveniencing anyone, you're just choosing not to buy something.

KNOW YOUR FACTS before you boycott something. Do your research to find out how a business is run, how its products are made, how its workers are treated, the impact it has on the environment.

Be vocal about why you're not buying a product – maybe it's environmentally degrading or unethical – and make it clear what the company needs to change to make it better. If you're young, others are more likely to listen. They'll be really interested in why you're boycotting and they'll want to be on your side to feel like they're making a difference too. This helps to spread the word far and wide, and puts pressure on the company to change its ways to avoid more negative publicity and so lose profits. Every news article, interview and social media post should help inspire more people to join the boycott.

As a young person you make a great 'human interest' story. Adults are often shocked when children and young people are informed and proactive and the story (small, helpless, innocent child vs. big, powerful corporation) is bread and butter to a journalist. Call your local paper or news site and tell them why you and your friends refuse to shop at wherever. Make it easy for the journalist – give them a photo opportunity by letting them know you'll be holding a demonstration outside whatever shop or HQ on a given day. Then be there with as many friends as you can persuade to come. Make sure you're clear about your message as well as being friendly and inviting so that other people will want to join in.

Boycotting is an extremely effective tool in pushing companies and organisations to change their practices, but that's not the only reason to do it. We all have some responsibility for this crisis, however small, and we need to question and examine our conscience in everything we consume. Could it have been made by sweatshop workers? Did trees need to be cleared in the rainforest to enable its production? One person refusing to buy a product with unsustainable palm oil in it may not make a big dent in a company's profits (though loads of people doing it will), but it will make a huge difference to your own responsibility for the crisis the planet is in.

I'm going to talk about some of the things that I feel you should consider boycotting or at least sourcing more sustainably, like clothes and palm oil, but I can't cover everything that has a negative impact. Once you start thinking about where everything is from and its cost and carbon footprint, you'll work out where you can make changes to better things and what you want to stop consuming altogether.

This is just a rough guide to some of the major things that have the greatest impact, things that people are already talking about and campaigning against.

MASS BOYCOTTS

Boycotting as an individual is easy in a practical sense, since it involves only you and your decision to stop buying or engaging with something. However, for that same reason, it can be hard following it through, and you may wonder how much impact you're making. Rallying other people and challenging in a more public way will make more impact and can actually be surprisingly easy.

There may already be a mass boycott campaign going on for something you want to challenge - like XR's fashion boycott - in which case you can combine your forces and work on getting the message to as many people as possible. However, you might not agree with the messaging of the campaigns that already exist, or maybe you want to focus on a different part of the problem, or a different audience.

NAME

KNOW YOUR

So I have a few tips for starting or growing a boycott:

As with an individual boycott, firstly know your facts. You need to be clear why you're boycotting a company or product and be able to justify your actions and defend them to the media.

The next important thing is publicity – you can't get people to join you if they don't know about you. Put pressure on well-known companies by naming and shaming and organize protests with banners and slogans either outside their headquarters or in really public and busy places. Remember though, if you choose an individual problematic

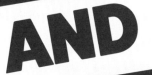

AND

SHAME

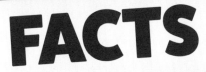

FACTS

brand or business to focus on, it's the company you're objecting to – the people who work there have families and lives outside of their jobs and no one deserves to be publicly abused or have their livelihoods threatened.

Create a Facebook event and blast it out on all the other social media platforms. Call the local newspaper or website and tell them what you're doing; if you can get coverage or an interview you can get your message out to so many more people. Write articles about the negative impact of whatever you're boycotting, publish them wherever you can, even if it's just online on a website you've made, and tell EVERYONE you know about what's happening.

Be really clear about:
– what you're saying
– why you're saying it
– what people should do about it
and get your facts straight – it will only make your argument/action/boycott stronger.

Start a pledge to boycott whatever you're focusing on and get signatures!

Don't be afraid to canvass on the street, even if it's scary initially. You might get a climate change denier – I did my first time, and I tried to talk to him for about a minute before I decided it was a lost cause, crossed the street and started canvassing there. It's a learning curve – it's nowhere near as scary the second time and you don't need to get it right every time. Just don't be fake with the people you're stopping, try to engage them and have a real interaction with them. You might make them stop and really hear what you're saying and inspire them to change their behaviour too. Give people a really clear message, backed up by

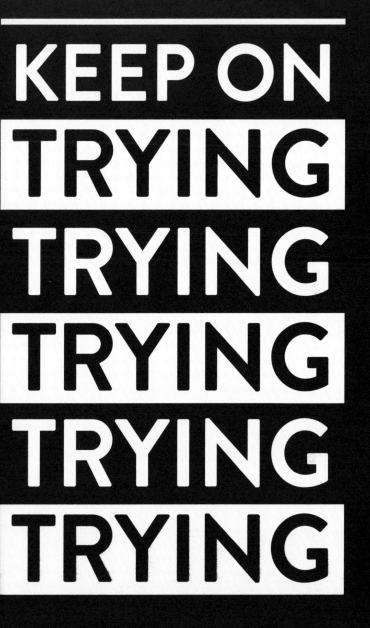

science and facts, but stay friendly or they'll become hostile and won't listen to you any more. You can't force people to change; all you can do is inform them and let them know the impact of their actions.

You could try to come up with original content – make a meme, something that's funny, that'll grab people and make them share it even if they don't fully understand the message behind it yet or even agree with it! The point is to go viral!

Even – or especially – if you're starting a new boycott, ally yourself with people who are already fighting. Even if you don't agree with their whole message, they may be able to give you a lot of advice and help, and we're all in the same fight. We all basically want the same things.

The environmental community can be a really supportive and amazing space to be in; you can learn a lot. Being in XR, surrounded by people who know what's happening to the world and are doing something about it, has been really good for me – especially in XR Youth where we're all going through the same climate grief and can support each other.

It doesn't matter if you get something wrong as you can always start again, try a different tactic, or ask someone for help. The point is that you keep on trying and whatever change you make, even as small as inspiring one other person to go vegan, will make a difference to the world. So go out there and get boycotting!

PETITIONS

HOW TO CREATE A PETITION

Petitions are a great way of showing that a number of people feel strongly about something without requiring much commitment from each individual or tons of organisation from you. They're a gathering of voices without having to physically get everyone together to a march or a meeting. And petitions make a difference! Even if you don't immediately get the result and numbers that you want, you'll have succeeded in putting your issue on the agenda and raising awareness of it. You'll have helped other people with the same concerns know that they are not alone, which will give them heart and may galvanise them to more action. And you'll have got a sense of people who you can contact or organise to further action in the future. So – what are the first steps?

DO YOUR HOMEWORK

Who is it you are petitioning? Who has the power to make the change you want? Your school? Your council? The government? Do some research so you know who makes the decisions and who to target with your petition. Find out how many signatures you'll need for them to consider it – most organisations or government offices have a policy on this. For example, the UK government will debate in parliament every petition with over 100,000 signatures – and respond to every petition with over 10,000.

KEEP IT SNAPPY

What do you want your petition to achieve – what is your goal? Don't focus on the problems – for example: 'People are using too much single-use plastic.' Concentrate on the solution – people will sign up to a call to action, for example: 'I call on the government to ban single-use plastic in this country by 2022.' Keep it short and simple but make sure you include what you want to happen, who can make it happen and by when. You can add a short explanation going into more detail about the issue and your feelings about it below.

PUT IT OUT THERE

If your petition has a local focus – for instance your school – take it out onto the street or other busy places like shopping areas. Although most petitions are now set up online, when it comes to the local community, face-to-face is best – especially if you want to target older people.

Make sure you have a lot of clipboards, pens and sheets of paper for people to sign. You might also want to hand out some printed sheets with information on your cause and what you aim to achieve with the petition. Get interested people to print their name and then sign, and also ask for their email address so you can keep them posted about the results of the petition. Include a tick-box asking whether they'd be interested in hearing about other actions you might organise.

For a wider audience, it's best to petition online. There are several global online platforms for change, including Avaaz.org, 38degrees.org.uk and Change.org where you can start your own petition. They take you through each step and have online support if you have questions – they make it really easy.

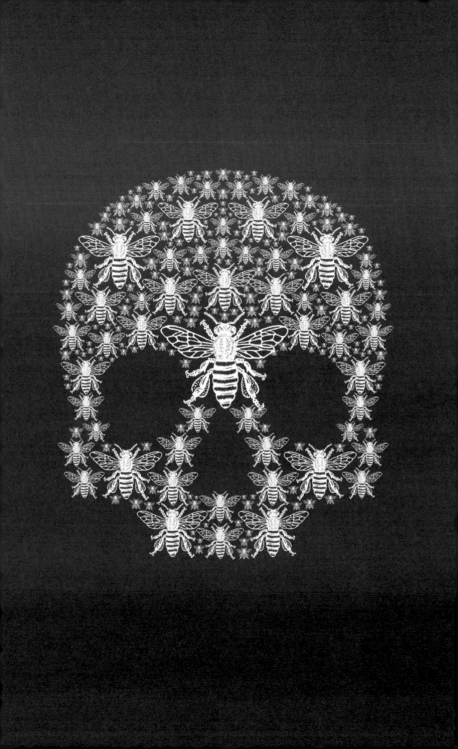

DELIVER IT

Once you've collected enough signatures, you can deliver your petition to the decision-maker.

First, ask them for a meeting. It might be best to do this on email, so you have a record of your requests and their response. If they agree, prepare what you want to say in the meeting and practise it so you don't get tongue-tied. Present the problem, say why it concerns you and then ask them to implement your request, and hand over the petition to demonstrate all the other people who are concerned about the issue and want action to be taken. Take pictures, post them on social media and notify everyone you can about the outcome of your meeting.

If your decision-maker won't meet you, don't worry, you can still deliver your petition. Invite the local media and tell them everything you would have told your decision-maker (who may look weak for not being prepared to engage with you). Take pictures and post them on social media and keep the people who signed your petition informed about what happens next.

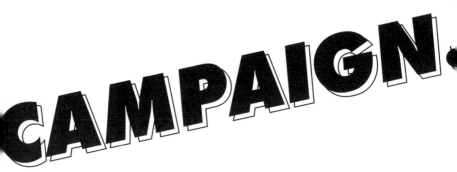

FASHION

There's been enough in the news about sweatshops and throwaway 'fast' fashion for it to be generally accepted that there's something wrong with the way the industry works and how consumers consume.

Fashion itself can be art – clothes and the way they are worn can be beautiful and meaningful, they can help you express who you are or want to be, and so make you more comfortable and confident. But much of the industry around fashion isn't about empowerment or art – just profit: how the most money can be made for the least investment.

Trends are a massive part of the industry, creating constant pressure for people to buy new things and then throw them away in an endless cycle. Although trends are nothing new, today they move much faster because there are so many different influences on fashion, from social media to catwalks and brands.

Many fashion companies sponsor influencers and advertise on social media to get their brands seen and talked about. And it's so easy – you can just click a link to get the exact same thing in your size. Video-sharing platforms are full of toxic clips of people buying huge hauls of clothing, alongside others of wardrobe clear-outs – people throwing out piles of barely worn clothing, just to buy more. Some boast on social media that they'll only wear an item once and then discard it.

Many fashion mass-producers are constantly churning out new items as cheaply as possible, often cutting out workers' rights and destroying local environments so they can provide ever-cheaper clothes.

But – good news – the fast-moving production lines can be easily disrupted if we just STOP. You can make a real impact and attract serious attention through boycotting unsustainable fast fashion companies. You could single out a specific issue, like paying workers below minimum wage or polluting rivers with dye-runoff from factories, and be vocal about why you're boycotting companies that do this.

Thrifting and second-hand shopping are being popularised by influencer figures like Emma Chamberlain. This practice

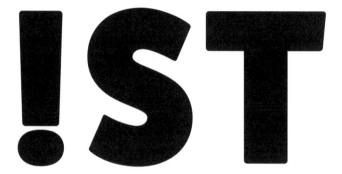

is much better than buying things first-hand – but even charity shops can have a negative impact. Anything with holes, stains or that even just needs washing may be thrown away and end up in landfill – as will most of the stuff that isn't bought within a couple of months.

There are other ways to get rid of your old clothes: on Depop or eBay, as presents or in clothes swaps with friends or organisations and apps like Swancy and reGAIN. Websites like the RealReal are also good, offering really affordable second-hand designer clothes, as well as luxury clothes made using textiles that have been responsibly produced and put together by craftspeople who are properly paid for their work.

Or try mending your clothes instead of getting rid of them, or repurposing them as rag rugs, blankets and curtains – the internet is full of tutorials on how to do this.

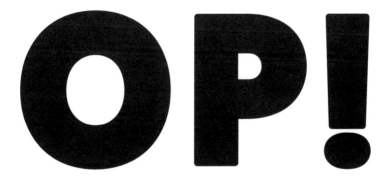

If you have to buy new, try to find ethical brands – some even offer warranties and will repair damage to their products. Even though these companies can be more expensive, in the long run you'll save money because the stuff lasts for so long. But be wary of brands that claim to be ethical and, for instance, recycle clothes. Recycling textiles is a largely untapped industry, with some start-ups trying out new technologies and attempting to combat the problems with waste. Generally though, not enough progress is being made to actually make this an economical choice for a lot of companies – so it's possible that any claim they'll recycle your old clothes is just greenwashing: an easy way to improve their image without changing the real issue of their toxic production line.

Fast fashion has been talked about a lot in the media and environmental organisations already – there are a lot of pledges and groups that you can join in with.

For example, XR has created a fashion boycott – xrboycottfashion.com – where you can pledge to not buy any new clothing at all for 52 weeks. This can be interpreted in different ways, from not buying anything first-hand – because even if you're buying from sustainable brands they're still making new things that we don't need – to not buying anything at all.

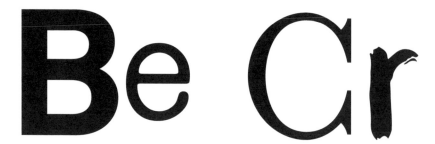

Instead of getting more stuff, you can save your money and be creative, figuring out new ways to wear items and DIY-ing old clothes. Take care of your wardrobe, don't wash your clothes every time you wear them. You really don't need to unless they smell – it fades and wears them out and it's a waste of energy and water. Learn to sew, patch and darn – visible patches can be beautiful and make the clothes way cooler too.

Whatever you do, try to be aware of what you're buying and what you're throwing away. When you start to really notice what you're consuming, you'll be able to tell what you need, what you'll actually wear, and whether you really need anything new.

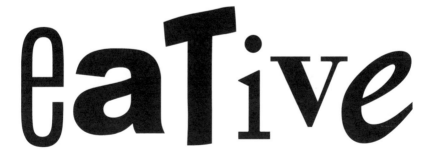

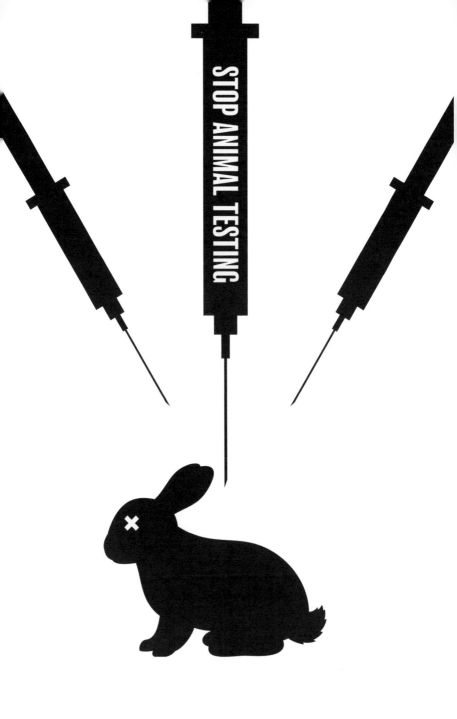

MAKE-UP

Although make-up isn't on the eco-radar as much as fashion, it can be just as bad in the ways it's being made and thrown away.

The production is often polluting and energy-intensive, with factories churning out thousands of increasingly cheaply-made eyeshadow palettes and lipsticks every day, usually packaged in single-use plastic that'll end up in landfill or the sea once the make-up's been used.

Huge amounts of waste from these factories also go into the local environment; the chemicals that many brands use in their products are hard to break down, so when they're thrown away they end up in lakes and rivers, leaking into the surrounding earth and eventually into the oceans and the food chain. Traces of chemicals relating to the cosmetics industry have been found in soil on farms and in household dust, which means that we're breathing air and eating food that's contaminated with potentially harmful chemicals.

The industry may appear to have solved this problem itself – there's a new trend for 'natural' products, with plant-based ingredients and fewer chemicals, but often the reality is that companies say they're 'eco-friendly' and natural but are using the same ingredients as before with a few natural ingredients added for branding. To make it worse, these natural ingredients may be produced on a massive and unsustainable scale, on land created by clearing rainforests, using pesticides and in monoculture systems, which destroy natural ecosystems. 'Natural' ingredients are also obtained using a whole host of unsustainable practices like mining for minerals – which may use non-renewable resources and cause air pollution, biodiversity loss, and water and soil contamination.

These policies may also cause human and animal rights abuses. For instance, mica is a glittery mineral sometimes used to add sparkle to eyeshadow or powder.

A 2016 article in *The Guardian* estimated that 20,000 children worked mining mica in just two Indian states. *Vice* magazine published another sobering article, reporting that an estimated 5-10 kids died in the Indian mines every month from accidents like collapses and also from lung diseases caused by breathing in too much silica dust.

Animal testing is also still a problem in the cosmetics industry. After the controversy surrounding it and several campaigns, a lot of companies are starting to produce cruelty-free products, but some brands are still behind the curve, continuing to use rabbits, guinea pigs and mice to test their products.

Taking all this into account, the best thing to do would be to stop buying make-up altogether. But make-up is fun and a really important tool for self-expression. I don't wear make-up every day, but I love putting it on for parties and when I'm in the mood. I have a lot of fond memories of experimenting with it with my friends and just by myself in front of the mirror.

This isn't me telling you that you have to give up everything in your life to live in the forest and eat berries. It's up to you to decide what you're going to carry on consuming and how you want to live your life. But I *am* asking you to consider your impact on the world.

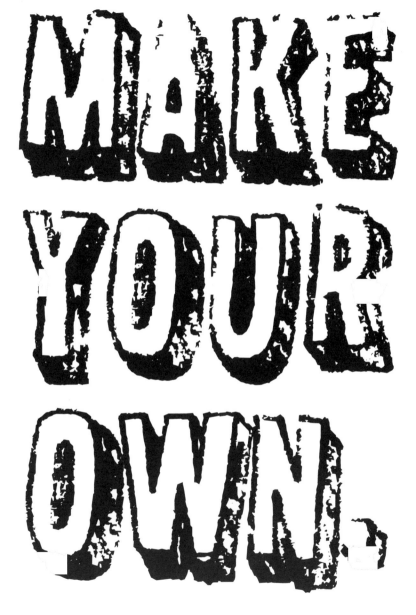

Some YouTubers and beauty gurus are popularizing no buy or low buys, where they buy fewer or no new cosmetics for a year and try to use the stuff that they already have, to avoid wasting it and to cut down on what they're consuming. If you do use your old make-up do ensure that it's safe to use and not past its best.

If you totally run out of make-up you could try making your own. There are tons of YouTube tutorials, and thousands of recipes online for skincare concoctions.

If you've got to buy make-up, at least research the company you're buying from and the ingredients that they're using. Try to find 100% natural, sustainable, biodegradable, vegan and cruelty-free products. Aim to have a scaled-back, minimal make-up collection with reusable packaging.

When it comes to taking it off, a flannel is always preferable to single-use wipes.

And don't forget to speak out against the most harmful companies.

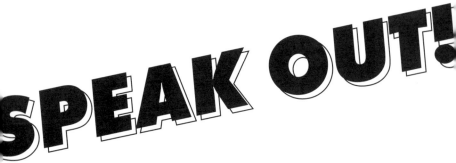

FLIGHTS

By now everyone knows that planes have a really awful impact on the environment. Taking one flight, even short haul (which means any flight of three hours or less), generates as much carbon as some people's total output over a whole year. But the demand has been growing, with record-breaking numbers of flights every year, prior to the coronavirus emergency.

People come up with all sorts of justifications and self-greenwashing excuses so that they can carry on flying everywhere without feeling bad about it. It's a mass self-delusional exercise, helped along by the media, publishing articles and promoting ads talking about 'the perfect holiday', which generally requires long haul flights.

The articles and ads are often accompanied by ways to supposedly cut your carbon footprint – like the e-tickets example (in the Intro); the same website also recommends going to the loo before you fly, as the additional weight of your pee will apparently make the plane use significantly more fuel. Attitudes like this are ridiculous, blatantly ignoring how bad flying is and the measures that we really need to take to make a difference. And seriously – if the weight of your pee causes so much environmental destruction that it needs to be flagged up, think of the damage your whole body is doing every time you take a plane.

Everyone feels they deserve a holiday. When you're constantly bombarded with travel pics on social media and people raving about how amazing their trip was, to be the one making the sacrifice when you know others won't is really annoying.

Sometimes it isn't even about the holiday – my mom's from America and her family still live there. We visited them once or twice when I was a baby, but we stopped going when I was a toddler because we couldn't afford it. A few Christmases ago though, we went to Texas because I didn't remember my granny. I was willing to sacrifice a flight's worth of carbon to meet her and I would probably make the same decision now. It's really hard to make these judgement calls, however, because you can end up just justifying everything.

The truth is that we can't afford to carry on flying. We need to cut down drastically, and we can't keep making excuses to do whatever we want regardless of the impact. A 2014 government study found out that 70% of the flights from Great Britain were taken by 15% of the population. A lot of people who can't even afford to fly don't get the chance to make a choice and the emissions from your flight will affect them no matter what. This isn't fair.

It's also annoying that alternative methods of transport that

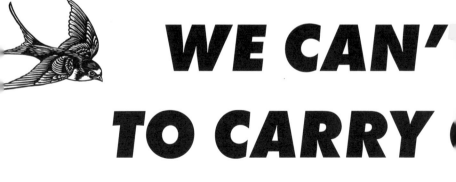

are greener are often more expensive. It often costs much more to travel by train than it does by plane.

A lot of charities and NGOs are trying to develop creative ways to stop people flying and to approach the problem from different angles. For instance, a classic reason to fly is that no one wants to waste precious days of their holiday on travel. One organisation, 'Possible', works on persuading companies to extend their employees' holidays so they can take the time to travel more slowly on boats or trains to their destination. A new Swedish campaign has persuaded 10,000 people to pledge not to fly for a year, the idea being that the hardest part is to break the habit and after a year of not flying you'll realise that you don't need to go on holiday abroad to be happy or satisfied with your life.

Others focus on carbon offset, offering to plant trees which will counteract the amount of carbon that your flight has put into the atmosphere. This is great in theory but offsetting isn't enough. We've built up such a backlog of carbon that even if we cancelled our emissions to zero right now, we would still have to be planting all the trees we can, just to start to get rid of the stuff we've already released.

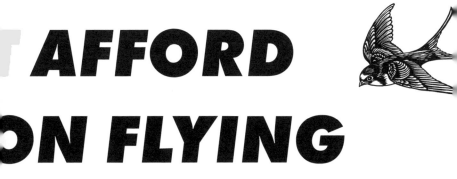

T AFFORD

ON FLYING

Offsetting can't be used as a free pass to release more greenhouse gases into the atmosphere.

The terrible COVID-19 pandemic of 2020 caused demand for flights to fall by 70%. This has made many people rethink the way they travelled in the past. Business people don't need to travel around the world to meet up when they can simply see each other on Zoom, Teams or one of the other video-meeting platforms. And many families are now communicating in the same way. Maybe we don't need to fly quite as much as we did in the past. Maybe we can do away with much unnecessary air travel.

If you decide to give up flying, you might meet with a lot of resistance. Your family might not agree with you at first. They might want to carry on flying everywhere, but if you stay firm and tell them why you don't want to fly they'll probably come around. At the very least, they can't force you onto the plane.

If possible, ask them to take the train or the boat instead, if it's affordable (but avoid cruises because many have more embodied carbon than the flight would). Ask them to go somewhere closer to home, like the countryside or seaside in your own country, via train.

Most of all, research the impacts of flying, and tell people what you find. Everyone who flies has to kick the habit if we really want to combat climate change. We can't afford to carry on jet-setting everywhere without a care for the consequences.

PALM OIL

Palm oil is an example of just how complicated and difficult it can be when you're trying to figure out the best things you can do for the environment.

Palm oil is super-useful in many industries. It can be found in around 50% of the packaged products sold in supermarkets across the world – from food to shampoo and other toiletry products. It's even found in biofuel.

Palm oil is cheap and easy to grow so with the logic of capitalism (if it makes money, it makes sense), farmers across the world have set up oil palm plantations. Large areas of rainforest have been cleared to make way for farms growing only oil palms – destroying habitats and creating a lack of biodiversity that means other plants, animals and habitats gradually disappear. Orangutans, tigers and elephants are among the many species threatened by loss of habitat. Much of the forest clearing is done by setting huge fires to burn the trees down, resulting in major carbon emissions. Along with the fertilisers and pesticides used in abundance on the plantations, palm oil production is polluting the water, soil and air of countries in Africa, Asia and Latin America.

These problems with palm oil have been in the media a lot lately (have you seen the Greenpeace ad with the orangutan? Look it up!) and public opinion even before that had started to shift against it. As a response, the industry set up its own standards to produce 'sustainable' palm oil. However, a lot of experts are saying that these standards are easily side-stepped and the sustainable label is often just another case of greenwashing. Many of the companies who responded to the backlash against palm oil with pledges to only use certified sustainable palm oil in their products didn't stick to their promise. At the time of writing, Greenpeace has revealed that some of the world's biggest brands are still buying palm oil from companies that destroy rainforests. They are sourcing from palm oil groups that are polluting and destroying ecosystems.

The obvious move, as with a lot of this stuff, is to boycott palm oil altogether, right? This could be hard, when it's in so many products at the supermarket, but it also might just make things worse. Some people suggest boycotting palm oil could actually increase deforestation and all the associated problems, as palm oil would just be replaced by soy and rapeseed oil, which may actually be worse because they are lower-yield crops, so they would need more land cleared to grow them and produce the same amount of oil. Then, there's also the possibility that even if you think you're avoiding palm oil, you might still be inadvertently buying it since some companies have chosen to rebrand it as 'vegetable oil', to avoid all the stigma that's becoming attached to palm oil.

By now you're probably tearing your hair out. It's tricky and complicated. You need to research it yourself to really understand all the different sides. I've probably missed something and there's new information coming out every day about the impact of this or that but I think, weighing up everything that I know, that it's better to buy products that are marked as having sustainably sourced palm oil, which at least is trying to set some standards and maintain them. It's a better alternative to soy and rapeseed oil and means thousands of people in the current palm oil industry don't lose their jobs.

Meanwhile you could try campaigning to get the sustainability standards raised and let people know about the corruption and negative impacts of the industry.

It's really hard to know who to trust, with companies greenwashing and governments turning a blind eye. It's why I don't want you to just take what I'm saying for granted - I might accidentally report a false fact or statistic. Challenge everything - including me. Research as much as possible. Fact check what people, companies, governments and the media are telling you before you believe them.

On a more positive note, there is an alternative to palm oil and other vegetable oil in development. Based on old NASA research, this alternative recycles carbon from carbon dioxide in the air to produce oils and protein. These are currently being used to produce fake meat and have the potential for so much more. New technologies are coming out every day and they may make a massive difference in the end. But in the meantime, we need to work on stopping the unsustainable practices first, as well as implementing new ones.

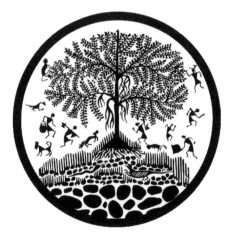

MEAT

My dad's a vegetarian, an environmental activist... and a sheep farmer. People are always confused by what seems to them to be a massive contradiction. His reasoning is that as long as there continues to be a demand for meat, he is taking some of that demand away from other farmers or producers who use worse methods to rear their animals and are causing more damage to the environment.

Our farm is organic and close to, although not completely, carbon neutral. It is definitely where I would want to live if I was a sheep. Obviously it's not perfect – they're still terrified of us because we gather them a few times a year to shear and dip them and give them medicines, and it varies but usually around half of the lambs are sent away to be slaughtered and eaten when they're old enough – but it's one of the most ethical and environmental ways of farming livestock, an inherently cruel industry. In my opinion if our farm shifts the demand from polluting factory farms, then it's doing a net positive.

When you look up 'animal industry pollution' or 'environmental impact of meat', there are pages and pages of websites about how eating meat is destroying the planet.

The UN released a report in 2006 that said the animal agriculture industry is responsible for 18% of all human-caused greenhouse gas emissions. This is a conservative figure and it's only growing. They found that the emissions weren't just from the widely blamed cow farts and burps, although these definitely contribute (methane has a much stronger effect than carbon dioxide (CO_2) at first because it absorbs heat in the atmosphere more easily, but it does break down much faster than CO_2). They're also from land deforestation for grazing, animal transportation, the meat-processing factories, the freezing and cooling and countless other parts of the process.

The World Bank says that 91% of the razing of the Brazilian Amazon rainforest has been for the animal agriculture industry. This clearing is getting rid of natural 'carbon sinks', releasing the carbon stored in the trees into the atmosphere while removing a means of processing CO_2.

These trees and ecosystems are not only being destroyed to create land to graze the cattle but also to create space to grow crops to feed them, which takes up a ridiculous amount of land. In fact, so much grain is being grown around the world to feed livestock that if everyone gave up meat right now, and all the livestock died of natural causes, we could feasibly end world hunger by giving the grain to people instead, and using the land that the livestock grazed and lived on to grow more grain and vegetables.

We would also save a significant amount of water if we didn't have to give it to the cows and sheep and chickens we rear for food. To grow the grain crops for the animals, added to what it already takes to raise the livestock, needs 15,000 litres of water just to produce one kilogram of beef. And yet more water is being polluted by the millions of tons of animal poo that leaks into rivers and lakes from the farms, making the livestock industry one of the biggest causes of water wastage and shortages.

All told, the animal agriculture industry is responsible for more environmental destruction than planes, cars and the whole transportation sector put together. However, there's not the same focus on its negative impact in the media and eco organisations. This seems strange, especially when

IT'S HARD TO JUSTIFY EATING MEAT

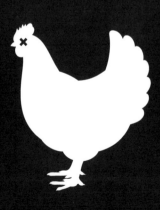

boycotting unsustainable meat producers or giving meat up altogether is such an easy way to immediately change the world...

It's hard to justify eating meat. Aside from the ecological impact, there's the morality of how many farming practices mistreat animals.

I loved eating meat and even when I learned about the environmental impact I didn't want to give it up. My parents love to tell the story of when I was little and saw a line of dead chickens hanging in a butcher's window. I decided then that I wasn't going to eat chicken ever again because it was cruel to kill them. But chicken was my favourite and my willpower failed immediately when that very night we had a delicious roast chicken and I couldn't resist a portion. I've always been good about knowing what my morals are and what I want to change about my habits but I'm bad at following through. Like many people, I'm selfish and don't have a lot of willpower.

It took a few years and a lot of guilt for me to become a vegetarian but I finally got to the point where I just couldn't justify eating meat to myself any more.

Diet is a really prickly topic with a lot of people because it's so personal and it takes a lot to change what you're eating. People get defensive about it; they don't want to feel guilty. You can't force people to stop eating meat or become activists – it has to come from them or it won't stick.

If you're going to carry on eating meat, try to find it from smaller local farms that are likely to be more ethical and sustainable. And if you can, try to eat grass-fed – or free range or organic meat where the animals are likely to have had a better life.

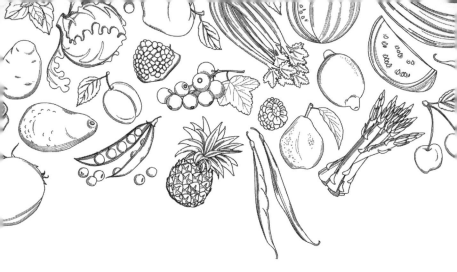

We live in a great time for vegetarianism and veganism. Most metropolitan areas are chock-full of vegetarian and vegan cafés and restaurants.

And the industry for meat-imitation products is growing: Greggs' vegan sausage rolls and Burger King's vegetarian burger are amongst those that have hit the media headlines. Of course the long-term goal is to rewild the cities, become self-sufficient and grow your own vegetables, but until that happens, a fast-food vegan burger is not the end of the world.

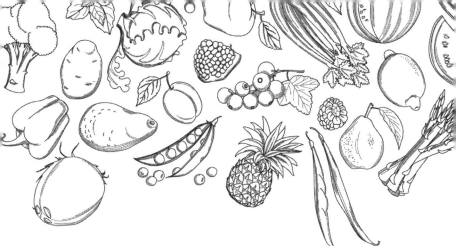

WE LIVE
IN A GREAT TIME
FOR VEGANISM

DAIRY (AND EGGS)

As I mentioned earlier, a huge amount of global greenhouse gas emissions are from the animal and animal by-product industries.

And the problems don't stop there. Much as with meat, a high volume of water is needed to make milk, cheese and other dairy products. More than 100 litres of water are needed to produce just one glass of cow's milk. The National Center for Atmospheric Research has conducted one of many studies which tells us that the planet is facing unprecedented drought in the next 30 years and beyond, due to climate change. It's possible that billions will die from dehydration, and we're still wasting that much water on a glass of cow's milk.

Then there's the perceived animal cruelty – forcing cows to reproduce every year so we can drink the milk meant for their calves. There are many reasons to consume less dairy, but for me it's mainly the way that the animal agriculture and by-product industry is destroying the earth.

I can't understand why some people are still refusing to even talk about veganism, saying things like, 'If we stopped eating them, farm animals would take over the world!' The argument I've heard the most is, 'You've eaten meat before in your life so you're a hypocrite and I'm not going to listen to you.' This makes no sense. It's unrealistic to expect everyone to have followed their current beliefs for their whole life, or never to have made mistakes.

We're all in different circumstances and under different pressure. We're all fallible. It's up to you to decide what your diet's going to be. No one can stop you from eating

GIVING UP DAIRY WILL MAKE A DIFFERENCE

WHICH MILK SHOULD I CHOOSE?

ENVIRONMENTAL IMPACT OF ONE GLASS (200ML) OF DIFFERENT MILKS

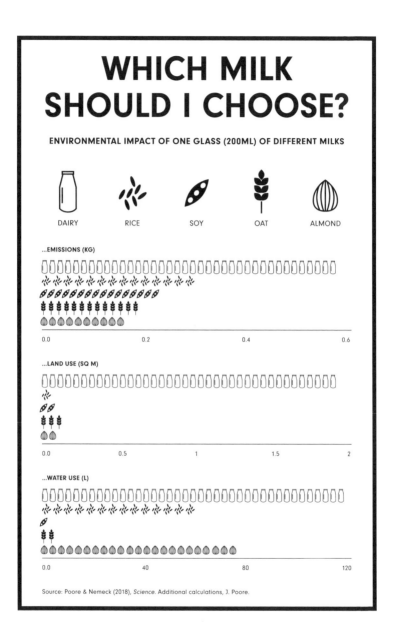

DAIRY   RICE   SOY   OAT   ALMOND

...EMISSIONS (KG)

0.0   0.2   0.4   0.6

...LAND USE (SQ M)

0.0   0.5   1   1.5   2

...WATER USE (L)

0.0   40   80   120

Source: Poore & Nemeck (2018), *Science*. Additional calculations, J. Poore.

whatever you want and the vast majority of vegans know this. The 'militant vegan' stereotype just isn't true – there are probably a few vegans who try to shame and guilt-trip non-vegans but no vegan has ever been rude to me about eating animal products.

So why are people so defensive about their right to eat dairy and eggs? It's like there's a wall in people's minds – they don't even want to engage with it as an idea and you often can't have a logical conversation about it. The only way that you can really talk to people about veganism is if you're not vegan, in which case you're called a hypocrite.

But if idealism is hypocrisy, how can anyone ever get better? For years I knew I should be vegan but I wasn't. Joining XR only made it worse, because a lot of people in XR aren't vegan and I was suddenly surrounded by people who were doing amazing things for the planet but still eating meat and dairy. This made me feel that my diet was OK and I could carry on consuming dairy. I've only just started trying to be a strict freegan (I don't want to contribute to the industry by buying any animal products, but I will eat them if someone is throwing the food away, if I scavenge it or bin dive for it, or someone else does, because I don't want to waste it once the damage has already been done). I'm still making mistakes but I'm trying and it's up to me to figure out how to get better. It's my responsibility.

Becoming a vegan comes with its own responsibilities. There are many vegan foods that are still bad for the environment. For instance, if you give up dairy for dairy alternatives you might still not be doing the best you could. Growing almond milk is very water-intensive and the soy crops for soya milk can contribute to deforestation. If you drink them you'll still have a negative impact on the planet

– but less than the impact the non-vegan foods would have had, so it's a start.

If you want to make a difference you have to start thinking about the effects of every part of your life. Giving up dairy will make a real change. Remember this isn't about some distant future generation. This will directly affect our lives and we need to change the future while we still can.

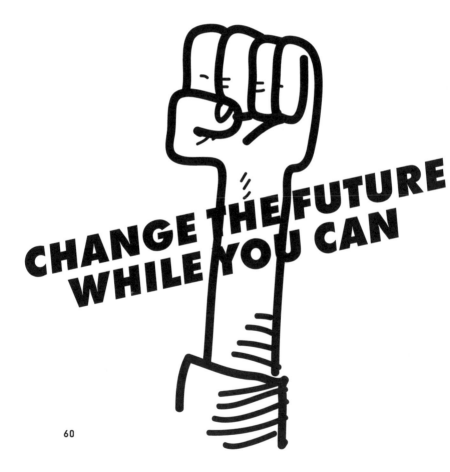

CHANGE THE FUTURE
WHILE YOU CAN

FISH

Fish could come under the category of meat, but I think the commercial fishing industry deserves its own section because some of it is really problematic.

A study published in *Nature* stated that between 1950 and 2003 our oceans lost 90% of their large fish like tuna, salmon, halibut and swordfish. That statistic is devastating. The demand for fish is so high that often they're being killed before they can breed, which destroys populations in the long term. These populations won't be able to survive for long unless we start to cut down on our overfishing; even then they might still be under threat.

The dredging and trawling techniques in wild fishing cause habitat destruction and water pollution. Not only this, but often the huge nets used endanger not just the target species of fish, but also the 'by-kill': the thousands of other fish and dolphins and sharks that are swept up in the nets and left to die. Many fishermen and women around the world aren't paid very much, so changing their techniques to save the dolphins isn't a priority.

It might seem that the solution is to eat farmed fish and leave the wild ones to reproduce and re-grow their populations, but farmed fish can be problematic too.

The farms take a lot more energy to run than just going out on a fishing boat, so they have a bigger carbon footprint than wild fishing. They can also have a bad impact on wild fish populations.

Fish farms are generally a series of nets positioned along a central walkway with an opening at the top, located in the sea or a lake. On many fish farms, each net can be crammed with fish, swarming together in small enclosures. The fish often develop diseases and parasites from being so close to each other and so may be given antibiotics to keep them healthy. However, the diseases they develop can spread easily through the water to wild fish, who don't have the same protection.

When you eat a fish, you're eating all the pollution that fish has been exposed to. Both a farmed and wild fish may have spent their lives ingesting the waste, toxic chemical overflow, plastic fibres and rubbish in our seas; a farmed fish may also have been pumped with antibiotics.

Farmed fish may also be fed smaller wild fish as one of their sources of food (which is also contributing to overfishing), so if you eat that farmed fish, through the chain you'll also get all of the pollution and diseases that the wild fish it's eaten have been exposed to. An example is dioxin-like chemicals (highly toxic compounds that are mostly a by-product of industrial processes) which leak into the water and therefore the fish. They're often found in higher concentrations in farmed salmon than in wild salmon, and linked to diabetes, infertility, heart disease and immune system degradation.

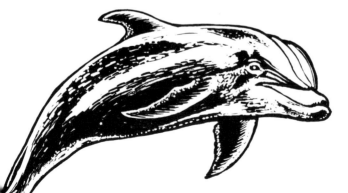

Many fish farms are approved by governments and local people as they give jobs to isolated coastal communities. I do think that it is important to support rural communities – I was brought up in one – but I also recognise that the fishing industry is a short-term solution. One estimate says that there may be no wild seafood left by 2048. Then the local fishermen and women will lose their jobs and only fish farms will remain!

Talking of my rural childhood, when I was nine, a fish farm was proposed off the coast of our farm and it was one of my first realisations that there was something wrong with how we're interacting with nature. My dad researched loads about fish farms and the effects that they have on wild fish and human health, but most local people wouldn't listen to him. They prioritised the extra jobs the new local industry said they would offer over the longer-term consequences, which is understandable from one point of view. As an environmentalist it's important to learn how to speak to people with different viewpoints. Maybe you can change some minds – just telling people what to do won't work.

Talking to people is great, but the most important thing you can do yourself is to cut down on your own fish consumption. If you're not prepared to give up eating fish altogether you do have some options. Make sure that the fish you eat is pole-and-line caught rather than net-caught or farmed. There are some companies out there that provide this.

You can also look up your fish on the Marine Conservation Society's Good Fish Guide. The website clearly explains population stock levels, methods of fishing and sustainability levels. It's a really useful resource.

There are many ways to campaign to preserve the oceans. You can boycott the worst fish companies and be vocal about the damage they're doing – join a campaign, like XR's Ocean Rebellion or the WWF fish campaign. You could try writing a letter to your MP or a celebrity, or you could tweet @ them. You could stage protests and marches outside company HQs or government offices or just somewhere central where there's a lot of foot-traffic. The choice is yours – but amending your own diet should always be step one.

YOU'RE EATING POLLUTION!

MY REVOLUTION STARTS HERE: *BUSINESS*

This is a section to note down your own thoughts. Are there any areas of your life you can change to make a difference?

Are there any products you feel you should boycott?

What makes them unethical or unsustainable?

How are you going to organise your boycott?

How often do you buy new clothes?

What do you do with your old clothes?

How can you reduce your clothing consumption?

_____
_____
_____
_____

How do you go on your holidays?

_____
_____
_____

Can you go flight-free this year?

_____

How can you convince your family or friends to go flight-free?

_____
_____
_____
_____

How sustainable is your day-to-day diet?

_____
_____
_____

Do you want to introduce veganism into your diet?

_____

If not, can you consume fewer animal products?

_____
_____

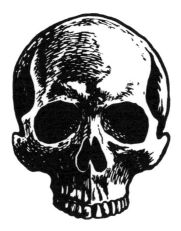

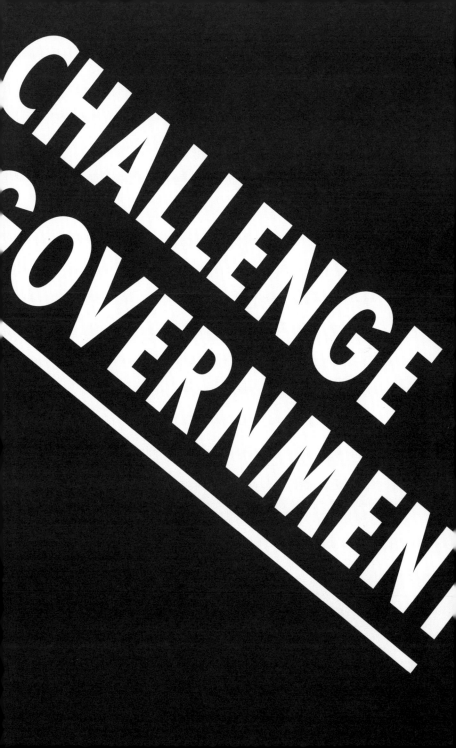

Activism is inherently political. By saying that there's something wrong with the world and no one is doing enough to fix it, you're also saying that there's something wrong with the system and the way that the government is handling whatever crisis is happening. People in power want to stay in power, so they don't like it when someone suggests that they aren't doing their job properly, especially in a voting country where they can easily be voted out of power if the electorate turn against them.

A lot of the last section about business comes back to governments enabling companies by allowing them to carry out environmentally-degrading practices, like fracking. Fracking is polluting to both air and water, among other dangers, yet the UK government only put a moratorium on it in 2019 – a temporary ban. If governments were actually on our side the climate and ecological crisis could already be solved with environmental laws and restrictions on businesses and carbon-intensive practices, but we haven't seen anything that will really make a significant change from most governments and ruling bodies.

This is disappointing because making them understand the situation we're in and successfully lobbying them to actually do something about it could be the only chance for our survival. Governments have a lot more power to make immediate change and to broadcast what is happening than individual citizens or organisations like XR.

As young people, we especially don't have a lot of political or financial power with which to lobby governments. We do, however, have a particular brand of emotive power. We're going to grow up in the world that adults make for us now, and we can hold them accountable for the world they're creating and what they're doing to our future.

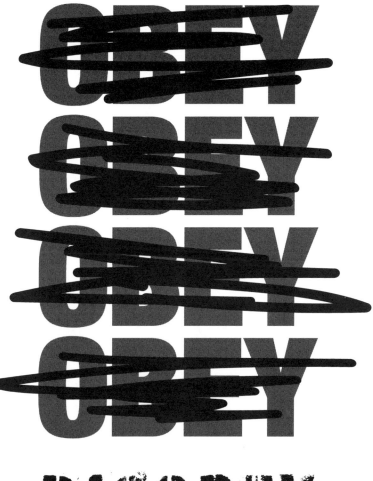

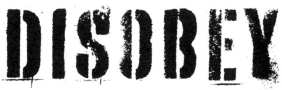

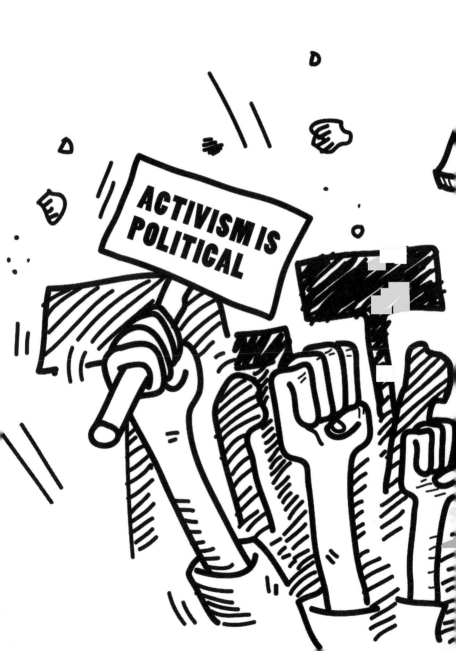

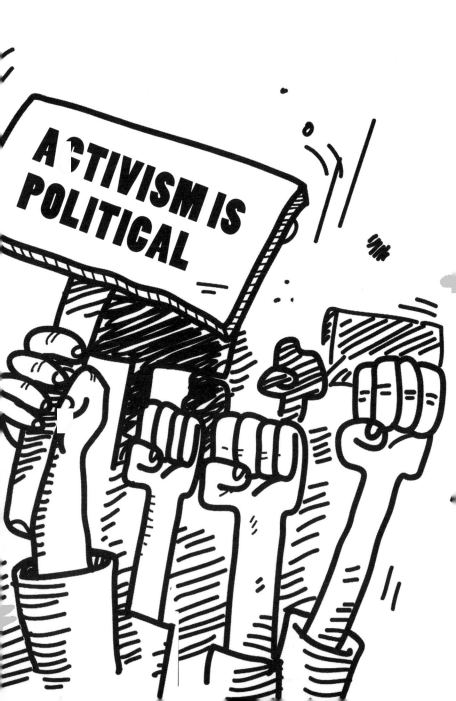

Pretty soon we're going to be the voters, or the revolutionaries: the people putting and keeping them in power, or not. We need to show them that we know what we want and we won't stand for anything else so that they'll change their policies and we can make sure that we and our children will survive this crisis.

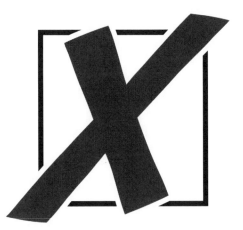

MAKE A
DIFFERENCE!

VOTE (IF YOU CAN)

This bit's simple: if you're old enough to vote (and lucky enough to live in a place where you can) then it's shooting yourself in the foot not to, especially as a young person. We're the ones who are going to grow up in the world being made by politicians now. We can't just leave it to the older generations to decide what happens.

If you aren't old enough to vote, educate yourself, decide who you support and tell people what your opinion is.

Old enough to vote or not, ask for others' opinions too as they might have another angle that you hadn't thought about or have more or different information. It's key to keep challenging yourself, and don't be afraid to change your mind. It's OK to not be sure or to decide that even if none of the options are perfect, some are better than others.

Even if you don't agree with your current political system, to me not engaging at all amounts to complicity. If you don't vote you're giving up a chance to actually make things better and stand up for what you believe in. In this case boycotting will make things worse, as it will mean that only the people who do agree with the system (and will therefore most likely have very different political views from your own) will be the ones with a say in what happens in your country.

Do your research, get out there, cast your vote and make a difference!

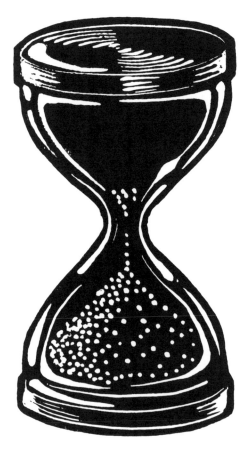

STRIKE FROM SCHOOL

The school strike for climate (Fridays for Future – www.fridaysforfuture.org) only started in 2018 and is already a widespread international movement that is making a real impact. School students take time off from class on Fridays in order to demonstrate and demand action from politicians and others to slow down, and hopefully reverse, climate change.

It began to really take off when Greta Thunberg mounted a protest outside the Swedish parliament in August 2018. She held up a sign that read 'Skolstrejk för klimatet' ('School strike for climate').

A global strike on 15 March 2019 gathered more than one million strikers and it's carried on from there.

The global school strikes have been super successful at putting tons of pressure on governments to start doing something and on schools to change their syllabuses and textbooks to educate pupils about the severity of the crisis.

I think that where the strikes are really making a difference, though, is in the publicity they get. They're raising a lot of awareness and getting positive attention. It's hard to tell kids to shut up and go back to school when they're protesting for their futures.

These protests can also be a way to get whole families behind the movement – most of these kids will be part of a family. If the adults can see that their kids feel passionate about the cause, they may take more of an interest than they might otherwise.

Going to a school strike has the potential to have a lot of impact (and it's really fun). It's just one day of classes you're missing so you can easily catch up.

Many adults aren't listening and so far seem to have ignored or been oblivious to much of the science and campaigns about climate change. However, the school strikes appear to have made a real difference in how people have started to view the issue. Now they're beginning to understand that it's about their kids and grandkids; that their actions may in the future subject us to drought, starvation and wars. They have a duty of care to us that they're realizing they aren't fulfilling. They have been leaving us to clear up their mess on our own but now they are finally starting to listen. People are responding a lot better to emotion than facts – we children have a lot of emotional clout right now.

I've been on permanent school strike for the past few months. I feel that this is the right choice for my life: I don't want to jump through the hoops any more because I believe that a lack of action on climate change might eventually cause societal breakdown. I feel that if we don't start seriously changing our attitudes I won't need the qualifications from school because our systems will have broken down totally, meaning qualifications will be worthless. However, it's a bit of a Catch 22 – if XR *do* achieve our aims and save the world, maybe I will need qualifications after all. However, it's a risk that I'm willing to take for a fight that I can't ignore.

It's easier for me than most, as both of my parents are very supportive, but other people in my life don't understand so much and I have to take a lot of time to explain my choices.

Not being in school, as well as being a form of protest itself, is giving me a lot more time to work on other forms of activism, like writing this book, taking part in more actions, writing articles and doing interviews to continue spreading the word and getting people to understand the severity of the situation. I feel like I'm not stopping my education, but choosing my own syllabus. I haven't stopped learning, I'm just learning about things that I feel are essential for the future of our planet.

However, I understand that what I'm doing isn't right for everyone – there's no one path that we should all take. After all, we need education of various kinds in order to produce the future climate scientists, people to research green energy and to engineer new sustainable futures. And we're going to need teachers, doctors, nurses, engineers and others. Learn in whatever way works for you – but make sure that you take action in your own way and that your voice is heard.

STRIKE!
STRIKE!
STRIKE!

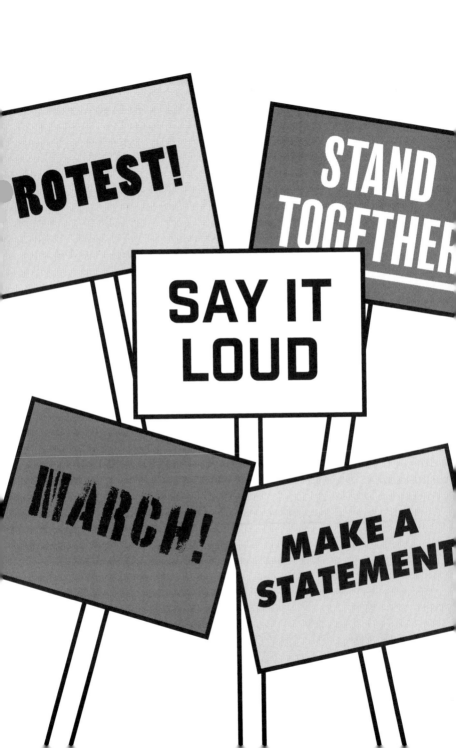

PROTEST!

Protests in one form or another have always been a cornerstone of successful social movements because they're a really good way to raise awareness of whatever issue you're championing. They're super media-friendly (journalists love to report from a protest – particularly a well-attended or unusual one) and also good for on-the-street outreach (getting the message out there to the general public), especially when they're in a busy or memorable place.

Protests are just one of the ways of making a statement, but they can definitely help to bring marginalised groups and issues to the forefront. They're an easy way to get more people to know about the problem and to stand with you and they can be used as a rallying point to inspire people. They can also build support for the movement so that more effective actions can be taken.

It's really important to see protests as a stepping stone to up the ante, rather than as a way to achieve immediate change. There's a bit of a guilt absolution thing that's often present in the environmental movement, where you go to a protest and then you drive home and have a steak dinner, feeling like you've done your bit for the environment.

Going to a protest is not going to magically fix everything. As well as shouting about it, we have to change our behaviour, what we consume and how we treat the planet.

That said, if there's a protest that you agree with, you should definitely go. You'll boost the numbers, especially if you share the news and bring friends, and you might get really good media opportunities to talk about why you're there and what you think should be done about the environment or whatever else you're protesting about.

Protests are fun. You can meet super-cool people who share your views and they're usually quite tame (at least in my experience in the UK, which might not reflect what happens in other countries – if you're worried, research what recent or similar protests in your country have been like). There's very little downside and a lot of positives.

Even if the protest isn't about what you're primarily campaigning for, you should still support other groups and movements. Sometimes groups that are working towards the same goal disagree about exactly how to achieve their aims. That's why I think it's important to recognise that we should all stand together and help each other. Creating unity and visibility for our cause across different organisations doesn't take much but it can achieve a lot!

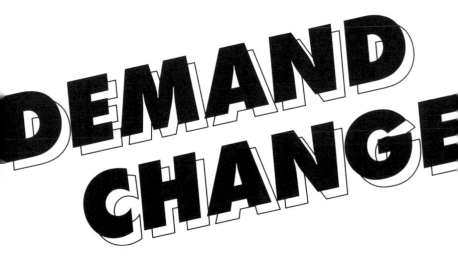

NON-VIOLENT DIRECT ACTION – NVDA

NVDA is a way of using your body to demand change, with actions like sit-ins and occupations, road blockades and strikes from school or work. XR uses a specific form called civil disobedience – purposefully breaking laws because you think they are unjust in order to make it impossible for people to carry on and just ignore you.

NVDA – and especially civil disobedience – gets results. In February 2019 there was a climate debate in the UK Parliament after the school strikes and very few Members of Parliament showed up. Then, in April, XR held the worldwide International Rebellion which saw activists all over the world demonstrating and closing down streets in major cities, getting news airtime and the support of the public. All this was done peacefully, using the guidelines of XR, to treat others with respect, help the emergency services and create a good, happy and supportive community environment. By May, just three months after the underwhelming 'debate', the UK government had ramped it right up and declared a climate emergency.

In May 2019 I was involved in the UK's first XR Youth action. Along with six other activists, I 'locked on' (chaining ourselves to railings) at a fracking conference. The UK fracking commissioner resigned a few weeks later, saying that their job had become impossible due to the government's concessions to environmental protesters. There were obviously a lot of things adding up to the resignation but I'd like to think our direct action was the proverbial last straw.

DISRUP

The police never even considered arresting us for that action, probably because we were so young. It looks really bad on them if they start arresting teenagers for protesting about their futures and there's a lot of extra process that they need to go through, like making sure there's a responsible adult present, so they're way less likely to arrest under-18s. Even if you're over 18 but still look young they usually err on the side of caution and avoid you.

Young people can generally get away with a lot more in direct action than older people because we're seen as less of a threat. I think, though, that we're actually more of a threat in terms of making an impact because we carry a lot more emotional power.

A few months ago I was at an action doing de-escalation, which means trying to talk to and calm down people who

TION
ACTION
GETS THE BEST RESULTS

are being disrupted by the action. A driver started shouting at me to get a job. I told him that I was 16 and in full-time education (which I was at the time) and he didn't know what to do, so he just took my flyer and closed his window.

Most of the things that people shout at you are just standard rhetoric; they don't actually think about it, they just say what they've heard other people say. If your comeback is simple and logical they don't know what to do and they usually just go away. Sometimes the only thing you can say is 'sorry' and hope they'll understand why you're doing what you're doing.

I do feel a lot of guilt for disrupting people who we aren't targeting. It's not our aim to annoy random people who are just trying to go to work, but disruption gets by far the best results and we're desperate.

Most people who are doing direct action don't actually want to be there. Sure, sometimes it's fun, but I'd much prefer to have a future and not have to be shouted at in the rain for hours. Right now I think that direct action is the most effective thing that I can do. I'm too young to vote and by the time I could become a politician or a scientist it would probably be too late. Also, protests and petitions aren't working. I'm not just going to let this happen and nor should you, so get out there and stand up for what you believe in. Let your actions speak for you.

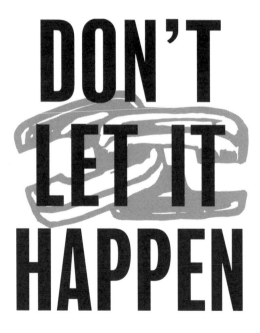

DON'T LET IT HAPPEN

GETTING ARRESTED – OR NOT

Part of the process of joining XR is deciding whether or not you are willing to become an arrestee. You must think carefully about your situation and whether your life can support your arrest.

Remember: you have to benefit from some sort of privilege to be arrested for your beliefs/convictions. For many people that sacrifice is not an option. Maybe they can't afford to take time off work or they have loved ones relying on them. Maybe they do not have permanent residency in their home country and can't risk their immigration status being compromised or even fear deportation. So if you put yourself out there in a situation that may end in arrest, remember that you are acting for many people who cannot. Don't take this decision lightly.

You also need to think about whether getting arrested will compromise your future prospects. Some professions may not be open to you if you have a criminal record, for example teaching or law enforcement, and this also may vary from country to country. So if you have your heart set on a particular profession, think carefully about whether getting arrested might affect your future.

I was arrested for the first time in the October 2019 International Rebellion. I was glued on to a structure in Trafalgar Square, London for hours before the police got me off and arrested me. It was one of the worst moments of my life. The police were shouting in my face. I was locked in a cell overnight (*the* worst night of my life) and that was where I spent most of the next day (my 17th birthday) as well. I didn't tell the police my identity at first. If I had, they would probably have treated me a lot better because I'm under 18. I thought it was more important to stand my ground and get as much out of my arrest as possible than be a bit more comfortable for 26 hours.

Although it was awful, and I wouldn't do it like that again, I'm proud of what I achieved. I was one of 1,300 people arrested in London over that week and as such I contributed to the global media coverage of the protest and therefore to more people learning about, understanding and joining our movement.

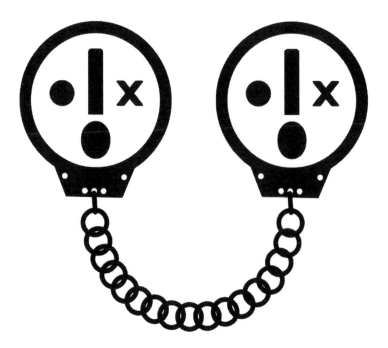

XR has numerous systems and structures in place to support arrestees. As with any action in XR, everything you do is done with your Affinity Group (see p.90) so you're never alone. On top of that, there's an Arrest Welfare Team that looks after us before, during and after arrest.

BEFORE

There are lots of clear, informative documents and infographics which explain your rights, what to expect when you get arrested and the consequences of arrest. These can help you make an informed decision as to whether it is something you're willing to risk for your convictions.

DURING

Every arrest is witnessed by an Arrest Witness rebel. These coordinate with Police Support rebels who stay outside police stations to greet arrestees when they are released. Being arrested can take a toll on your mental health, so emotionally it's very important to see somebody who shares your ideals and understands the struggle when you are released.

AFTER

A telephone network of Post Arrest Liaisons (PALS) offer emotional support and help with the logistics regarding court appearances (accommodation, travel, etc).

HOW TO PLAN
A DIRECT ACTION

When I first joined XR I didn't know how to plan or carry out direct actions but I soon got the chance to learn from lots of experienced people around me. I also had the opportunity to try things out and sometimes get things wrong so I could learn from my mistakes.

Activists are usually highly skilled, highly educated and highly organised. The general public and the media may often see activists as people who just want to disrupt because they don't fit in or can't be bothered to 'get a job', whereas their skills mean that many of them could walk into all sorts of senior roles in other organisations. It just so happens that they want to use their talents to make a difference to society and the world.

I'd really recommend joining your local XR/XRY group, like me. It'll mean that you can see the ways that experienced people organise actions and you can learn from them. It'll also make it much easier for you to find people to help if you want to do your own actions – especially people with useful equipment like trucks and rigs or trailers. You'll meet super-cool people of all ages, make friends and start new communities as well. Most XR Affinity Groups have been formed from non-violent direct action (NVDA) trainings in local groups.

XR Affinity Groups are small – usually fewer than ten people who take part in NVDA together. Affinity Groups are really integral to decentralised actions as they mean that there are small groups who know each other, feel comfortable together, cover each other's backs and do more direct actions. It's really important to have a team. Don't do it all on your own as you'll end up really stressed and burnt out and the action probably won't be as good as it could be if you work with a team.

Direct action isn't necessarily civil disobedience – it doesn't have to be illegal, although it will often make more of an impact if it is. If you're worried about pulling something off, for your first couple of actions try doing small and legal things so that you can get experience. It's important that you, and whoever is organising the action with you, figure out how to work together and safeguard yourselves and anyone else on your action before you try anything more high-risk.

The most common actions that XR does are lock- or glue-ons. These are where activists lock or glue themselves to something in order to disrupt. The targets of these actions range from public places to company HQs or even making roadblocks. Often these are combined to create maximum disruption and to generate even more attention.

Swarming (short repeated roadblocks – very low risk of arrest, but the public often get aggy), sit-ins and die-ins (symbolically 'dying' to make a point) are also widely used. You can also be really creative, for example putting on theatrical performances which are, of course, legal. The sky is your limit! Also don't be afraid to copy and adapt past actions – it's fine to repeat them. Sometimes repetition is how a message sinks in! Just make sure that the messaging still holds and you agree with it.

The messaging is a really important part of every action, and everyone taking part needs to know exactly what it is.

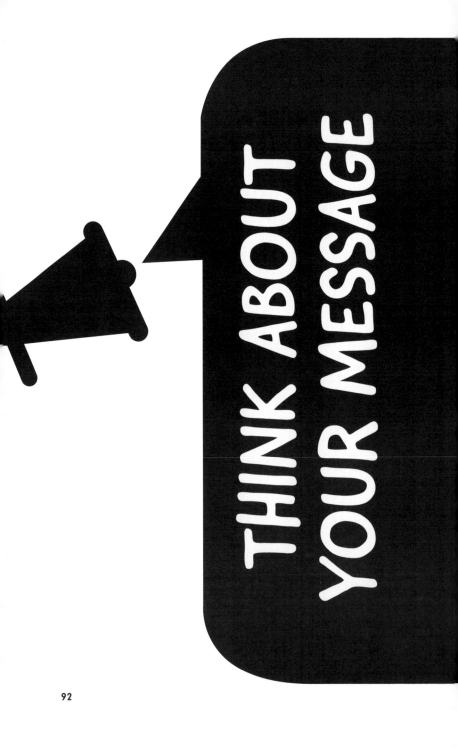

When planning a direct action, think about:
- Your MESSAGE - what are you trying to get across to as many people as possible?
- Who or what are you targeting - are you aiming at government, polluting companies, the general public?
- Why are you doing what you're doing? This will ensure that your message is clear. Where are you? What is the symbolism? What are your demands? What are the facts?

Make sure you have Bustcards. These are available from greenandblackcross.org and provide you with key advice, information on stop and search and arrest, and the names and numbers of solicitors who can help you. It's also recommended that you write the name and number of a solicitor and a protest support line on your arm.

Make sure you know and spread the five key messages:
- No comment (you don't need to answer police questions - stay quiet)
- No personal details (you're not required to give these under any stop and search legislation, unless you aren't a citizen of the country you're in)
- Under what power? (ask the police under what power they are proposing to charge you)
- No caution (don't accept a caution without asking a solicitor - cautions are a way the police will try to get you to admit guilt)
- No duty solicitor (use a recommended solicitor with experience of dealing with protesters).

After an event is over, it's important to get your team together and debrief. This means everyone reporting on what happened from their point of view and discussing what went well, what went badly, and what could be improved. We call these roses, thorns and buds.

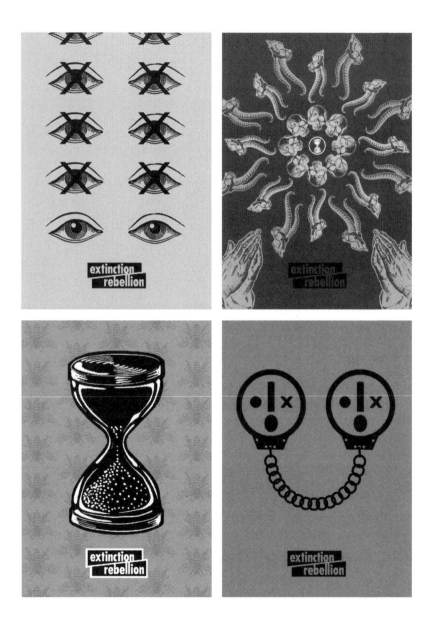

PAINT THE STREETS

'Paint the Streets' was a week-long mass action started by XR in the run-up to the International Rebellion of April 2019. Its aim was to get the word out about the Rebellion and XR by posting messages about it in the physical environment rather than just online or on bits of paper.

Activists used:
- posters (fixing them with wheat paste – you can find recipes online)
- stickers
- stencils
- paint that they applied to roads and buildings (using non-toxic paint that will wash off over time).

Art can grab people's attention in a different way from simply preaching. So long as property isn't damaged this is a great way to get a message across. It can be beautiful, provocative and thought-provoking and declares XR's presence in a new and stimulating way.

It was so successful and became so decentralised that it has never stopped and people are still doing Paint the Streets actions in their local Affinity Groups around the world.

It's become common practice after a meeting to grab some posters and go out flyposting with everyone or to do some on the way home with your friends or when you're bored. I always carry round a bunch of stickers to put on the bus or at train stations and whenever I have a marker pen I turn the ads on the trains and buses round so you can just see the plain back and write things about climate change on them. It's a bit fiddly but you get the hang of it. You should try it!

I think Paint the Streets is more a state of mind than an action. It is about creating art and spreading awareness about climate and ecological collapse, making something beautiful that will reach people and make them understand what's happening.

It's not just limited to flyposting; Paint the Streets covers street art, murals, performances – even busking and stand-up poetry. It's basically the idea of making so much art that it's unmissable so that everywhere people turn, they'll see artful expressions of our message.

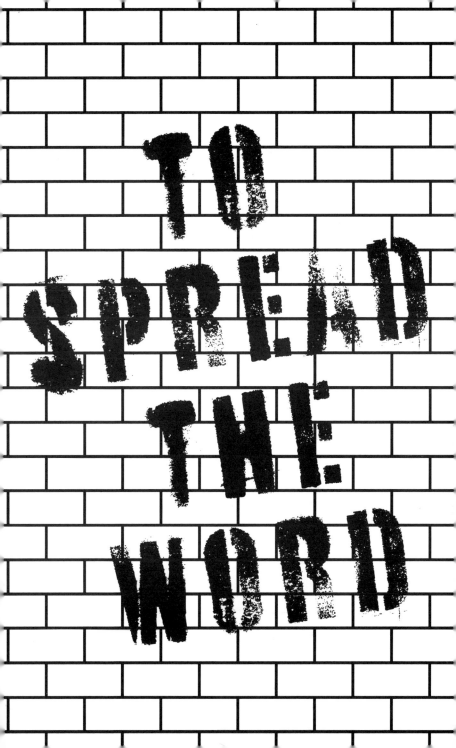

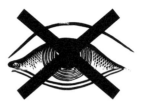
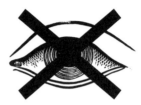

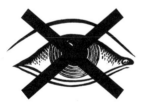
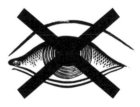

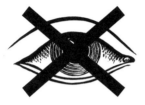
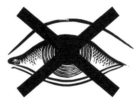

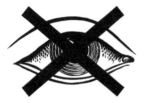
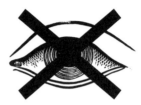

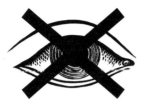
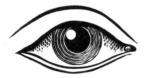

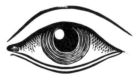

FIVE WAYS TO TALK TO A CLIMATE CHANGE DENIER

You may be doing an action in the street or talking to your auntie but chances are that you're going to come across someone who says that climate change is a load of rubbish. In that kind of situation, your mind can just go blank but here are some things that may help:

1.
STAY CALM, RESPECTFUL AND KIND

You will not persuade someone by rubbishing their opinion or making them feel stupid. If they respect the way you handle yourself and your approach towards them, your own conviction may sow the seed of doubt in their mind over time. People are unlikely to want to lose face by admitting that they have had their opinion completely changed on the spot. They are much more likely to think about your comments and information and may even repeat it to others in the future if you take this approach rather than being confrontational or preachy.

2.
TRY TO FIND COMMON GROUND

There are things that you are both worried about – for instance floods, forest fires, health concerns. If you can explain how climate change leads to something directly affecting the person you're talking to, they may be more ready to listen and understand.

3.
GET YOUR FACTS STRAIGHT

It is a fact that the overwhelming majority – probably 97% – of climate scientists agree that global warming is happening and humans are causing it. So even if there is the odd scientist (very odd) who claims that's not true, who are you going to go with? The ninety-seven doctors who say you should treat a deadly disease, or the three who say 'go ahead, you'll be fine'?

4.
FIND THINGS YOU AGREE ON

However, facts and figures rarely change people's minds – they usually have their own to fire back at you and it just turns into fact tennis. You could both agree that no one can say for certain what will happen in the future and then discuss the hypothetical possibilities. Examine the best and worst possible scenarios that may play out if climate change is real and if it isn't.

Let's say we do act against climate change and it turns out it isn't real after all – we spend a large amount of money and waste it, possibly causing a worldwide economic downturn. But if we do act against climate change and it turns out it IS real, we did the right thing.

Let's look at the alternative. If we don't act against climate change and it isn't real after all, we do fine. If we don't act against it and it IS real, we face not only massive economic worldwide depression but also an entirely different world. A world with constant 'natural' disasters (caused by humans) where floods, droughts, hurricanes and tidal waves become the norm rather than an exception. A world where our food sources from agriculture, farming and fishing are compromised leading to famine, global health pandemics and the breakdown of societies, leaving us with no way to get back to what we had before.

Hmmmm. If we look at these possibilities, it seems to make sense to take precautions against the possibility of the biggest risk. In the same way that a doctor cannot guarantee that bad things will happen if you continue to smoke or you don't get that dodgy mole checked out, you still probably know you shouldn't risk it. So why take that risk with the planet?

5.
THE LAST RESORT.

Lastly, you can always point out that climate scientists are humans too and no human would want this to be true. There is no motivation for them to lie about predicting the end of life as we all know it.

MY REVOLUTION STARTS HERE: *GOVERNMENT*

What are your political beliefs?

_____
_____
_____
_____

If you're able to, do you vote? If not, why not?

_____
_____
_____
_____

Would you consider striking from school?

_____

Would your family and friends support you if you did?

_____
_____

What would you say to them?

_____
_____
_____

What protests have you been on?

_____
_____
_____
_____

How did they affect you?

How did you contribute to them?

Have you ever spoken to a climate change denier?

If yes, what did you say?

If not, what would you say?

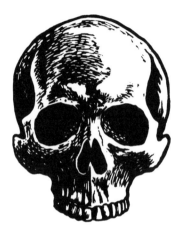

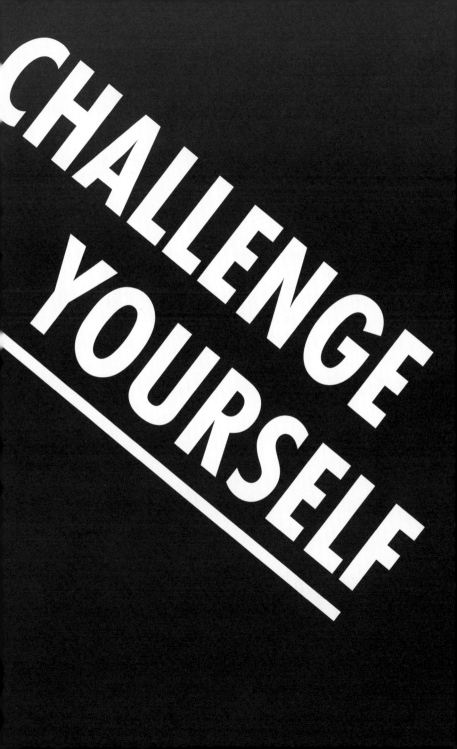

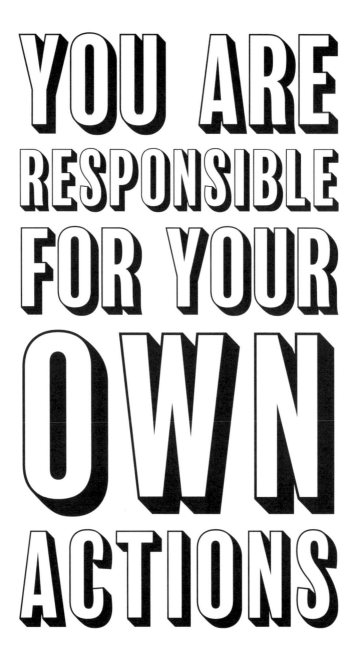

If there's one thing I want you to take from this book, it's this: YOU ARE RESPONSIBLE FOR YOUR OWN ACTIONS.

You can't just hide behind adults and blame them for everything because not everything is their fault. We've all contributed to the climate and ecological crisis, knowingly or unknowingly.

Every time you take an Uber, go on holiday on a plane, buy new trainers, even turn on the lights and heating, use the internet or watch something on Netflix, you're contributing to climate and ecological collapse. You're directly contributing to the destruction of rainforests, wildernesses and the extinction of humans and many other animal species.

You don't have to do anything that I talk about in this book but there is no escaping the stone cold fact that you're responsible for a part of what is happening in the world and you will make things worse if you don't stop to think about what you're doing and cut down on what you're consuming.

The fact that almost everything you do is destroying something is a fact I'm really struggling with and I know other young people are too. We've been thrust into this toxic society where adults tell us that we can do whatever we want and don't need to worry about anything but that's not true.

If I was given the choice right now to not know about climate change, I think I would take it. I don't want to be consumed by this, protesting and disrupting people and getting arrested. But I do know about it and I can't give up and do nothing. That's the burden of our generation - we have to live with the guilt, the knowledge of what our actions are doing to the world. And we have to fight.

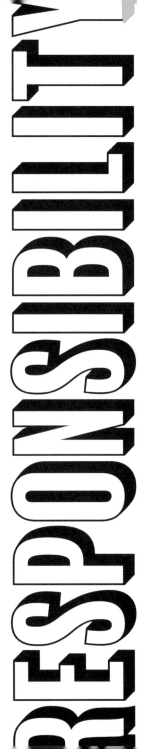

RESPONSIBILITY

We can't have the same complicity as those adults who think nothing can be done and therefore do nothing, ignoring science and the suffering of millions of people just to carry on normal lives. That's not an option for us.

In the Western world we're not yet dealing with the effects of climate change in the same way as in some other parts of the world, but it is a matter of time.

Something has to be done to prevent the future wars, genocide and starvation that we'll all be caught in. We have to give ourselves the chance to survive. If we carry on as we are now, we don't have any chance and we're condemning innocents – future children, animals and ecosystems – along with us. We all have to change how we're living but more than that we have to change how we're thinking.

You have to change your mindset. You have to start listening to evidence. You have to educate yourself and reconnect with the world around you before it's too late and it's all gone. And even then, if you survive, you'll need to be able to fend for yourself and build a new world.

SELF-SUFFICIENCY

Here's the hard truth: societal breakdown is a distinct possibility if we don't figure out how to stop and reverse climate change.

Drought, famine and disease might become the norm and everything you know now and that seems normal to you could change completely. Without enough food and water our whole system could break down. There might not be any power, because no one would be in the power stations working, so there might be no electric light or heating. Petrol stations wouldn't work so there'd be no cars, there may be no police or law enforcement because the government may have collapsed, or it might have turned totalitarian. It is likely that the richest and most powerful will be able to avoid the worst of it – the elite are already building their bunkers – but for most of us, it's so important to learn self-sufficiency.

If this situation does happen, you won't be able to rely on anyone else to do things for you so you must learn how to do them yourself.

In order to survive in a climate apocalypse you'll have to know how to build a fire, how to mend your clothes, how to defend yourself and how to forage. You'll need to find out what plants you can eat and which ones you can't, and also how to grow your own food. But you don't have to learn these things on your own. You can skill share with friends, or go to bushcraft classes.

And these skills can be applied to your life today to lower your carbon emissions and therefore do your bit towards preventing this apocalypse from becoming a reality.

If you grow your own food, you won't be contributing to food miles or adding pesticides to the environment. If you learn to cook, you can cook your home-grown food, or buy loose veg at the market in order to feed yourself, which means you won't have to rely on plastic-wrapped supermarket fruit and veg or prepared meals. Mending clothes means having to buy less.

Learning new skills can also give you things to do that aren't as polluting or carbon intensive – find a hobby like gardening or a sport instead of watching TV or Youtube or going out shopping. These new activities will also make you happier, as spending time outside is proven to improve mental health, so get out there and try something new!

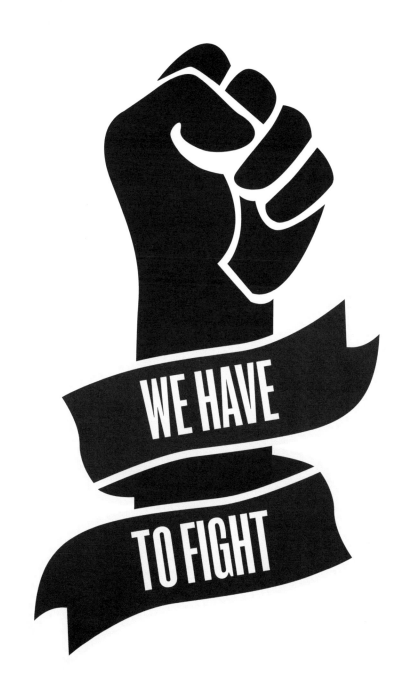

QUESTION EVERYTHING

It can be hard to trust governments and the mainstream media. Everyone has an agenda. It seems it's often all about gaining or staying in power for politicians and selling more papers and advertising for the media. Too much of the media is owned by too few people who are promoting their own views and opinions. That's why I think you should question everything – don't just trust and accept the things that you are told.

Think about something you might consider to be a fact. Why do you believe it? Is it because someone told you or because you saw it in the news or on Google? Even if someone you trust told you, do you trust them to verify their sources and know that what they're telling you is fact? They could have read it online, or someone that they trust could have told them.

If everyone was rational, they would look at the evidence, consider the options and pick the best course of action.

Unfortunately, very few of us are rational. We all fall prey to fallacies and biases but there are ways that we can make ourselves less susceptible.

Think about what you're taught at school, what are considered to be the necessary information and skills to prepare you for life. Who chooses these? And what life are they trying to prepare you for? The life that society thinks is an appropriate one for you, a life that serves the way things are at the moment. Think about this in the selection of your education, what it covers and what it doesn't. Some stuff is useful. For example, from history we can learn from the past. But is the history we are being taught useful? Are we being shown examples from the past that serve the present? I wasn't taught a lot of history, and even what I was told was exam-based and largely centred on the West. There's no historical precedent for the climate and ecological emergency – at least in recorded human time – but there are other examples in history where facts have been ignored, such as the two World Wars, leading to disaster. Can we learn from them?

Rationality and logic are things that a good education should teach, as well as a thorough and unbiased understanding of other people's cultures and religions, and what their morals and beliefs are. We need to understand others and challenge our prejudices and things like in-group bias in order to build an ideal society without discrimination. Understanding other people's ways might influence your own understanding of yourself. If you agree with a tradition or moral from another culture, you might decide to adopt it as part of your own moral code.

It's also useful to have an understanding of psychology, mental illnesses and trauma and why people believe what they do, the fallacies and biases and traps we all fall into. How we're influenced and manipulated by companies and advertising, governments and individuals, and how to see through them and analyse everything for ourselves.

Find out about the injustices in the world, the organisations working to save people and plants and animals, the intersectional struggles – like the impact the climate crisis will have on immigration and refugees – and how to help.

You can find this stuff in books and online and from people you trust. Mentors come in handy here. If you don't have one (or some) I would highly recommend finding someone to help teach you. They don't have to be older than you or fit into any preconceived mould of 'a mentor'. You can tailor the relationship however you want to, just find someone who knows about a subject that you don't, who can teach you and help you to understand and grow.

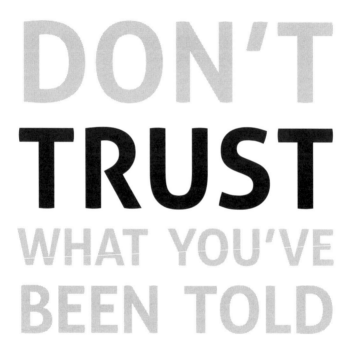

DON'T TRUST WHAT YOU'VE BEEN TOLD

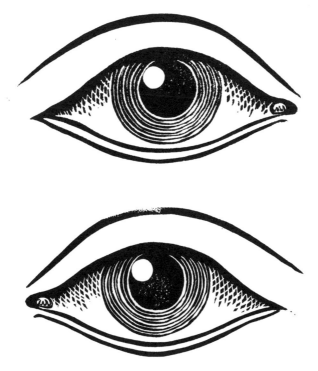

DECIDE YOUR OWN MORALS

A part of educating yourself about the world is also identifying what you believe in and what you think is right and wrong. We're often taught in broad strokes, bad or good, but things are more nuanced than this. There's a lot of middle ground out there!

Our morals have usually been inherited from the religion or society in which we grew up. For example, most of us accept that stealing is bad because we were taught it as a child. We didn't examine it and decide that it was morally wrong ourselves (although, on reflection, I think we can agree that in most instances it's not very nice). Identifying your own boundaries is an important part of growing up.

Right now, many countries are in an interesting place. There are a whole host of different religions and beliefs in many societies, and we're lucky that many countries are diverse and tolerant. This is a good thing because people are able to decide their own boundaries. We can understand the moralities of different cultures – we're not just stuck believing what our own families believed.

Some have turned to the law as a moral compass. They believe that if something is illegal then it is automatically wrong. This is flawed, as most laws weren't created for moral reasons, they were created to keep people under control. It's also dangerous. If the law is always moral, then it can never be changed, even if it's discriminatory or out of date. The law must evolve and develop as society changes.

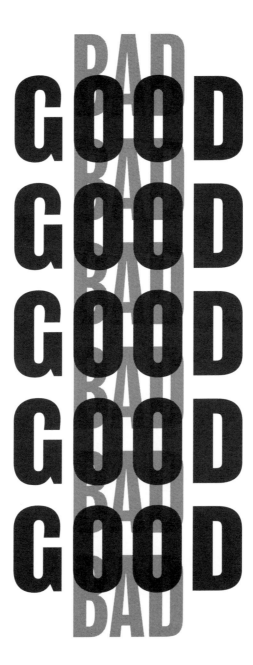

You need to decide for yourself what your morals are. Find a mentor and talk to them about it. Don't ignore other people's morals and set yours in stone – be flexible. Change means that you're growing and developing your ideas and you aren't going to get stuck with a flawed moral code.

Personally, my moral code keeps me going. It gives me the impetus to fight for the natural world, especially when I'm not feeling up to it some days. My moral code guides me to tell the truth in order to save the people, animals and plant life that are dying or will die from climate collapse.

What does your moral code do for you?

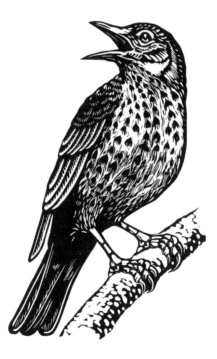

YOU MAY BE YOUNG, BUT YOUR OPINIONS ARE VALID

It's really important to know that your opinions and ideas are just as valid as everyone else's, even (especially) people older than you, and you need to trust yourself to be able to hold your space. People can be ageist, both against the young and the old, but their perceptions can be altered and it now feels like change is in the air.

As young people we need to start holding space and talking about what we want for our future, rather than leaving it all to adults who have a very different perspective from us. Not all adults are the same of course – grown-ups are also speaking out about the climate and ecological emergency and doing it for their kids, and future generations, not just from a sense of survival. But they're still in the minority and we need to change that.

A lot of it is about bravery. It's scary speaking up. I've experienced older people tittering when I have something to say. It's important to ignore behaviour like this, to not care what they think and speak loud and clear. Your message will resonate – it will find a home.

As young people, speaking up is necessary for our future. We have to do this because we're the ones who'll suffer when there's a climate apocalypse. We should have a say in the decisions being made and the way this battle is being fought. We should have some influence on how our systems are going to be run.

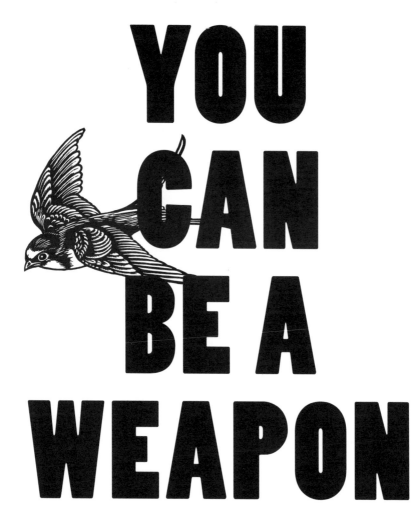

YOU
CAN
BE A
WEAPON

The mainstream media have often been really resistant to platforming stuff about the environment so we need something really big and impactful to encourage them to cover it. Maybe protests are too accepted nowadays. They're legal if you get a permit so no one will really care about what you're doing unless you get massive numbers, which is hard.

You need a good angle to attract serious media attention, something new that people haven't necessarily seen before, and we, as youngsters, are in a position to provide this and give a fresh perspective. Take XR's Red Brigade. They were created by a UK street performance group, The Invisible Circus, from Bristol. The group appears dressed all in red with their faces painted white so they look like living statues. The group often perform mime or create tableaux during XR demonstrations. The red symbolizes the common blood shared with all species. It's an amazing sight to see.

Being a young person can be a powerful weapon in the media. The emotional side of being young in the climate crisis can be really good for reaching people and attracting attention and publicity. Many won't expect young people to be clued up enough to talk about this thing that most people are ignoring or don't even know about and when you know the facts, it'll throw them.

But more than that, we're in an awful position. Our futures have been stolen from us and we need to do all we can to raise awareness of the situation.

Don't be afraid to speak up!

LEAVE

TO

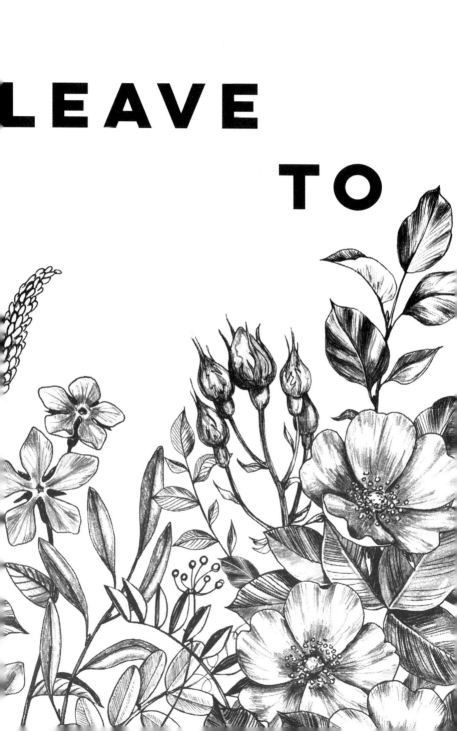

THE WILD
RE-GROW

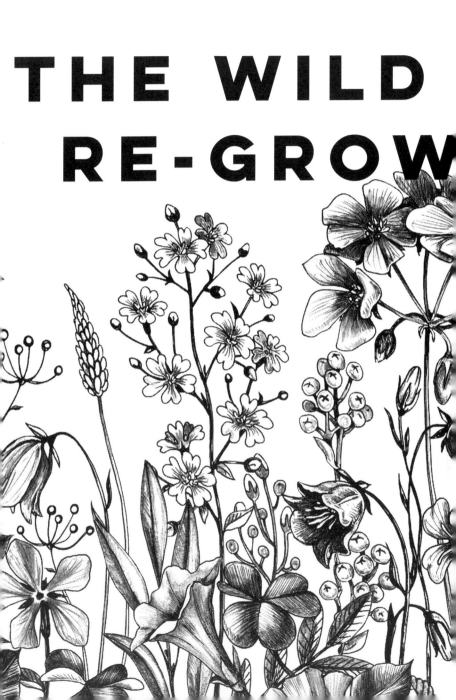

RECLAIM, REWILD, RECONNECT

Communities are much harder to create without somewhere to meet and it's hard to find a place that's free – or at least cheap enough. But actually there are so many places in every city that aren't being used – old buildings, abandoned pubs, hotels and churches. You can claim these spaces and squat in them, or, if you're very lucky, you might be able to track down the owner and persuade them to let you use the space until they develop it.

Sometimes spaces that are supposed to be for the community aren't actually being used – like the little green squares in fancy neighbourhoods that you never see anyone in. And kids used to play games in the streets before there was so much traffic. In fact, we saw some good examples of reclaiming the streets during the COVID-19 pandemic – cars gave way to socially distanced street events such as clapping for the health services and carers, musical performances, keep fit sessions, dancing, and more.

In the XR April Rebellion one of my favourite moments was when we played football in the street in Marble Arch in London, which is usually choked with cars. Also, on Waterloo Bridge we had stages for music and poetry, a kitchen and a beautiful garden with trees and flowers, and even a pond. There was music and dancing at all the sites and I saw how much space is being taken up by roads and what we could do if there weren't any cars, or many fewer.

Reclaiming space isn't just about squatting or occupying it for yourself, it's about finding a use for it for the whole

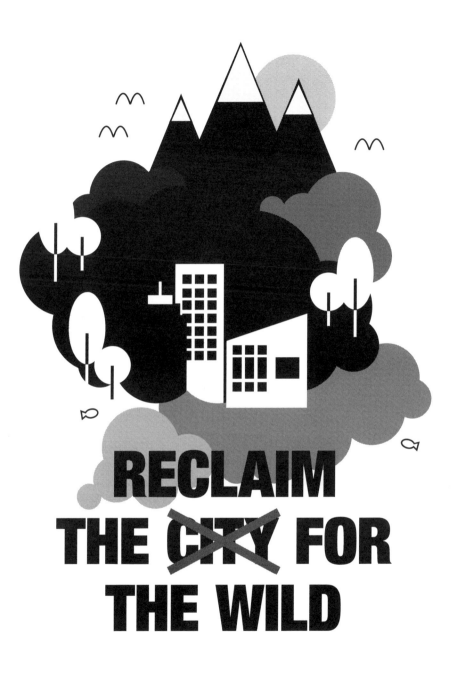

community, such as planting trees to make it green and holding events for everyone. Start guerrilla gardening in your neighbourhood – plant herbs and veg wherever you see space, or if you want, you can talk to the council and see if they'll approve you doing it. They might even give you a grant. The people on my street got permission to have trees all the way down the pavement and we all got together and planted them with flowers around the base of each tree.

I've grown up in some of the wildest and most remote countryside in Scotland so I was in nature for a lot of my childhood, but I've also had the counterpoint of living in one of the busiest cities in the world so I've really seen both sides.

When I started getting involved in XR and all of the climate change information suddenly got real for me, I started to break down. I couldn't deal with all the grief and pain and guilt. It seemed like there was nothing I could do and I could feel myself sinking into a hole of depression and fear. I was really homesick, something that I'd never really felt until then. I went on a Reclaim the Power camp (look it up!) and on one of the days I ended up just being alone in the countryside. It was the happiest day I'd had for a long time. All the problems and walls that I was facing seemed less important and I could just be in the moment, climb a tree to pick some plums, go swimming in a lake, chat to some dog walkers. I felt like a massive weight had been lifted – I needed to be out of the city, in nature.

When you're in a city, it's easy to feel disconnected from nature and the countryside. Instead, it's easy to become blinded by consumerism, with ads and shops telling us that we need this or that product, that it'll make us happy

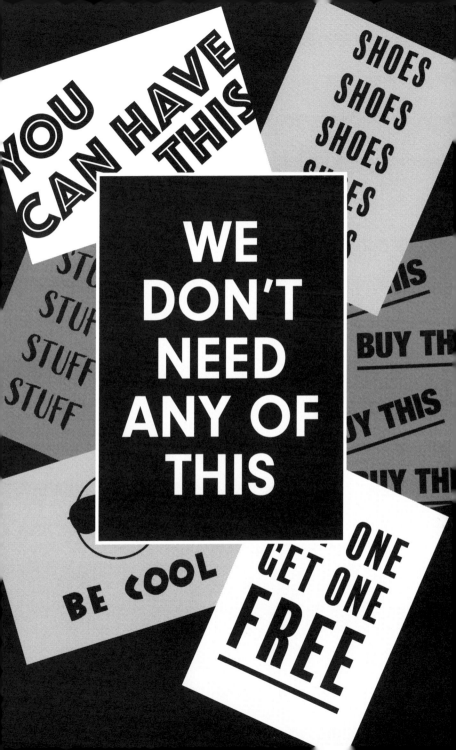

and fulfilled. The truth is we don't need any of this crap – we'd be much happier and more fulfilled with genuine interactions, relationships, and the freedom and peace of the wild.

One of the effects of the COVID-19 lockdown was the fact that so many of us shopped less, bought less and reconnected with our families, friends and with nature. We slowed down and appreciated the smaller things in life.

I was very lucky to have been able to go to the Reclaim the Power camp. Being able to leave the city and go to the countryside is a privilege, and not everybody has the time or money to do so. Luckily there are open spaces filled with wildlife even within the confines of most cities.

So find a space with nature. Somewhere quiet and peaceful. Somewhere you feel free. Go for a walk. Climb a tree. Go swimming. Look at what we're destroying if we carry on as we are. Look at what we stand to lose.

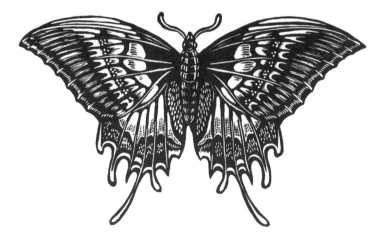

SCAVENGING

My mom is almost magical in the way that she can find things by rummaging through charity shops or identifying unloved objects through friends, or even finding things on the street. If you ask her for some trainers, she'll find some in no time.

Scavenging sounds unattractive but it's such a good way to get things sustainably and to cut down on landfill waste. It's also way cheaper than buying things new, so you save money and often get things you wouldn't have been able to afford anyway. Things that someone else is chucking out.

I define scavenging as a number of different methods of acquiring what you want without buying new. It's not just bin-diving and getting things off the street. It's also using charity and second-hand shops, hand-me-downs from friends and family, apps like Olio and TooGoodToGo and freecycling. It's going around food shops and bakeries and markets just before they close to see if you can get any of the food they didn't sell that day. To me, scavenging is pretty much anything that involves taking and re-using pre-owned stuff or food that's going to be wasted and thrown away otherwise.

Even times of celebration can put your scavenging skills to the test. My family are experimenting with having an eco-friendly Christmas this year. We're doing stuff like not using any heating, so we wear boiler suits and jumpers to keep warm. We have a little potted Christmas tree that someone gave my sister last year that we're going to decorate and we've decided not to buy any presents new and to get creative instead.

I've been scouring junk shops for stuff for my friends, doing paintings and drawings and buying experiences, like theatre tickets and train tickets to the countryside. Last year my mom pioneered hot water bottles that she makes from our old moth-eaten jumpers. They were so popular that she's making them again for everyone that didn't get one last year. And my sister is doing all my dad's darning for him. It can make for more rewarding gift giving. Something that someone has spent time and thought on is so much nicer a gift than something they grabbed the day before Christmas Eve, no matter how much it cost. So get creative at Christmas!

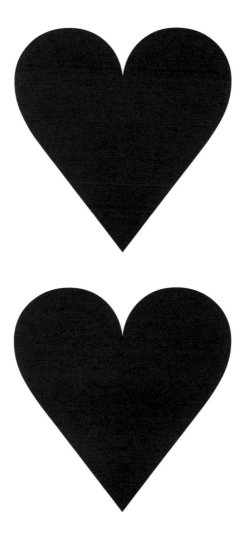

HOW TO EAT

We sometimes forget that everyday acts can have a big impact on the environment. Take food – we often mindlessly consume without paying any attention to how the food reached our plate. In earlier sections I talked about meat, fish and dairy but even if you're vegan do think about where your food is from. If you're eating avocados and jackfruit from far-flung countries, think about the air miles that they've travelled. You might be feeling smug about your choices, but the pollution involved in transporting foods over many miles and continents is a big problem.

Eat local and seasonal. Eat fruit and veg when they're in season in your country and you're not only helping to save the planet but also they'll taste better – they'll be fresher and more full of flavour. There are also a number of restaurants and cafés that are sustainable (minimal or no waste) and serve food sourced locally (often within just a few miles). Find out about them and if your family are having a celebration suggest going to one.

And how about trying to grow your own? If you have a garden, great! Research seeds or buy plants that have been grown in your area – or even better get them from friends – and get growing! If you have a balcony or a window box, equally great! Sow seeds in boxes or pots and soon you'll be harvesting salads, veggies or fruit. If your local area has allotments, suggest that you share one with your parents or friends, get your name on the waiting list and you can grow a whole host of things. Allotments are often very cheap to rent and you'll save lots in food bills. Or in some communities, guerrilla gardeners have sown herbs and vegetables for the community to use. Follow their

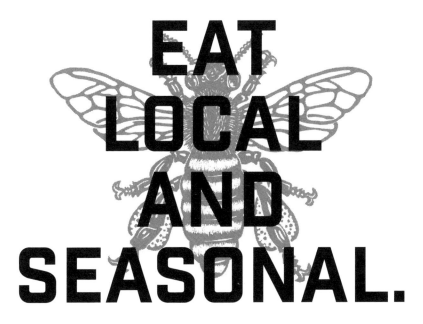

EAT LOCAL AND SEASONAL.

example in making a space more green and beautiful, and providing a source of food for yourself and others too.

Growing your own produce also means that you will encourage local wildlife – lots of plants attract insect pollinators, and if the birds and other wildlife steal a bit of your produce it won't matter. Just tell yourself you're helping to keep them alive and supporting natural diversity. And there are even foods you can grow with no outdoor space at all and just a pot on a windowsill. It all counts – and it's fun. It also helps you to reconnect with nature and appreciate the natural cycle of the seasons and how plants grow.

Eating locally is not limited to fruit and veg – try to support local businesses but always find out where their raw ingredients are coming from. The ideal is a local supplier who uses local raw ingredients of course, but the fewer food miles your dinner travels the better.

Making your own cooked food from scratch is also more sustainable than buying ready meals or takeaways. There's far less packaging or processing, it's likely to be better for you, and home-cooked food is less likely to contain palm oil and other problematic ingredients. Learn how to cook, use local ingredients and do your bit.

You can also use technology to cut food waste. There are apps that help households and businesses to donate surplus food rather than throwing it away. One such app is Olio, a free website that helps you to give your surplus supplies to other local people – if you're going on holiday or have bought or grown too much, for example. There are lots of others – just search for food waste apps.

Here's to us all making an effort to grow and cook delicious and healthy food and help to save the planet in the process!

COMMUNITY

Humans are social creatures. A community is a group of people who know, love and support one another emotionally and in other ways. A community can achieve what individuals alone cannot because it pools together lots of different skills. You may have a friend who is very good at writing, another who's a great public speaker and another who's an artist. Together these skills can complement one another to achieve great things. This can be seen in activism.

Community is important because the young generation today seems more isolated than previous generations. A lot of people talk about our generation being the 'social media generation' and they are not wrong – we love to be online. This comes with positives and negatives. Sometimes it increases loneliness – being online all day every day means that we are disconnected from our surroundings and from other humans. Sometimes however it is the conduit towards finding our own communities – we can befriend people from all over the world through common interests.

There is a mental health epidemic today in young people. Lots of loneliness, depression and anxiety are exacerbated by the issues of our age. Fear of the climate crisis, racism and the rise of the far right are often made worse by the influences of social media and cyberbullying. To combat these fears and worries, your community can offer support.

Family can be important. In Iceland the government found that when they gave families vouchers for group activities, it encouraged them to spend more time together, which then positively affected the mental health of the teenagers of those families.

It should be acknowledged that not everybody is lucky enough to have the support of a loving family and even for those who do sometimes it's not enough. Western culture doesn't promote living with an extended family, and it can be so great to be close to your aunts, uncles, grandparents, godparents, family friends and more. That connection is something that most young people really miss out on.

Inter-generational relationships can be an important learning experience – even if you don't always see eye to eye! The old and the young have much to learn from one another. We need a community, a support network, to teach us how to build relationships and make sure that there is always someone to support us. If you aren't close to your grandparents or no longer have them in your life, I recommend volunteering some time to work with older people. There are so many stories to be heard – and you can talk to them about the climate crisis too.

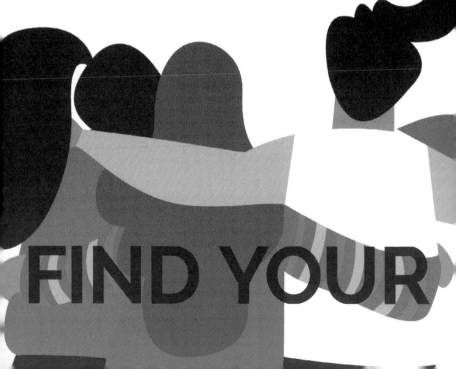

FIND YOUR

Whether you're close to your family or not, the modern world allows us to make our own community elsewhere. Sometimes communities can crop up in unconventional places. One of the best I've experienced was in a squat in North London, in an old hotel. The people who lived there were trying to create a safe space to build their community and they all cooked meals and ate with each other. Whenever I went to the squat I felt like I was in a really incredible supportive space – totally unlike any I've been in since.

The closest I have to a community is XR Youth. We're all going through the same climate grief and struggles that many others in our lives don't understand. They've supported me through a lot. I encourage you to find your support network – find your tribe.

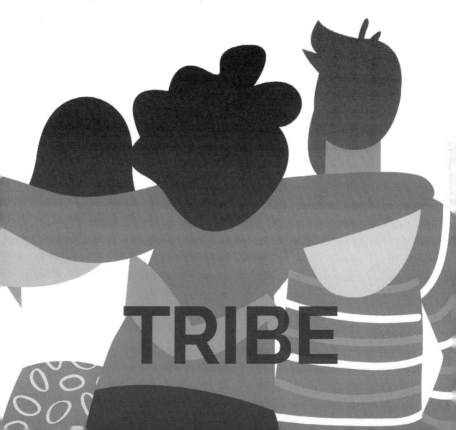

TRIBE

 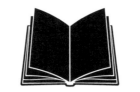 

 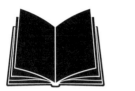 

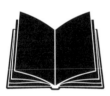 SUPPORT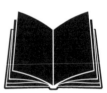

YOUR

 LIBRARY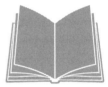

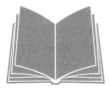 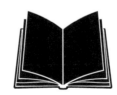 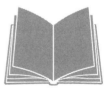

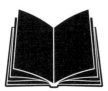  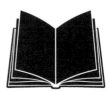

CONSUME ART

What do you want to consume? How do you want to spend your time and money?

Each time you spend money, you make a value judgement. You decide that the thing you're buying is more important than all the other things that you could get for that price. The same value judgement is true of the environmental impact of whatever you're buying – you need to weigh up if the thing you're buying is more important to you than any detrimental environmental impact it has had. For example, is your shampoo more important than any rainforest that's been cleared to grow the palm oil ingredient?

My dad always says that art is a product you can consume. Instead of consuming gadgets or trinkets, we can consume literature and poetry, music and paintings. Spending your time and/or money accessing art will significantly reduce your footprint because you're not spending that time and/or money on more carbon-intensive activities. Galleries and libraries are havens in our consumerist world. Support them. Not only will you be supporting the planet but you will become happier. Buying something new may give you a thrill for an hour, or even a day, but I really think that nurturing an appreciation for art will make you happy indefinitely. Art is emotional. Through it you can have a real human connection, feel what others are feeling and learn from them.

There is an argument that sustainably produced books are carbon sinks, which means that they hold more carbon than they release and prevent it from going back into the atmosphere. This is because trees absorb carbon and are then cut down and made into books. It's a beautiful idea that objects that transfer ideas and knowledge also contain carbon. Especially if you get them from the library!

If you have a creative streak, then make art yourself. XR has its own art group that make our protests look fantastic. Getting together with like-minded artists to make powerful banners, posters, placards and more is a great way to contribute to the movement.

Which brings me to my next point. As well as consuming art, you can also consume company. As well as making art, you could spend your time going to the park with friends or making them a meal instead of going out to eat or getting a takeaway.

Another option is to have a party! We don't have enough celebration in our lives, and you can reclaim spaces and build communities with parties. You don't need to pay to go to some fancy festival, or go to a club where they have overpriced drinks and you might not even get in if you're under age. Find an excuse to celebrate, put the music on and dance!

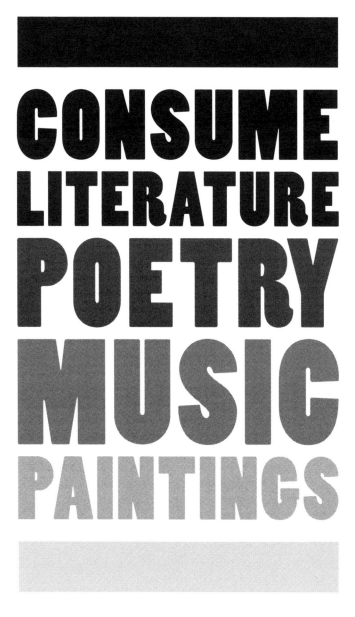

CONSUME
LITERATURE
POETRY
MUSIC
PAINTINGS

MY REVOLUTION STARTS HERE: *MYSELF*

How can you cut down on what you're consuming?

In which areas of your life can you consume less?

Which communities do you consider yourself a part of?

What do you value about them?

Do you have a mentor? Who do you look up to?

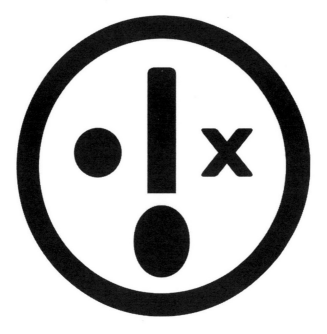

So, that's all I have to say for now. There may be contradictions in this book (nobody's perfect), but I think it's clear we all need to start acting – fighting – for the future. Because if we don't campaign, protest, boycott, and do everything possible to make a difference, there will be no future (for us humans at least).

Resolve to do all you can to make a difference.
Research and know your facts.
Have an opinion.
Make your voice heard.
Do *everything you can* for the survival of the planet.
The future is in your hands.
You can make a difference.
Fight.
Challenge everything.

How do you spend your free time?

Are there any ways to make your hobbies more sustainable?

Are there any ways that you could experience nature more?

What skills should you learn in order to be more self-sufficient? For example sewing, cooking, growing things, repurposing possessions?

